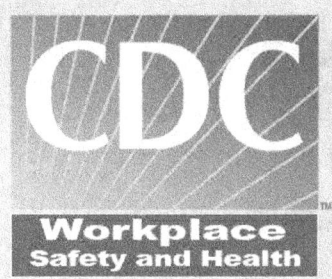

Evaluation of indoor environmental quality at an accounting office

Rachel Bailey, DO, MPH

Chris Piacitelli, MS, CIH

Stephen Martin, Jr., MS, PE

Jean Cox-Ganser, PhD

Health Hazard Evaluation Report
HETA 2011-0096-3176
Florida
April 2013

DEPARTMENT OF HEALTH AND HUMAN SERVICES
Centers for Disease Control and Prevention

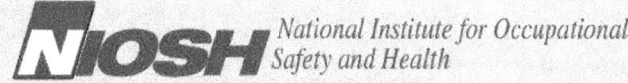

National Institute for Occupational Safety and Health

The employer shall post a copy of this report for a period of 30 calendar days at or near the workplace(s) of affected employees. The employer shall take steps to insure that the posted determinations are not altered, defaced, or covered by other material during such period. [37 FR 23640, November 7, 1972, as amended at 45 FR 2653, January 14, 1980].

CONTENTS

ABBREVIATIONS

μg	Microgram
AHU	Air handling unit
ANSI	American National Standards Institute
ASHRAE	American Society of Heating, Refrigerating, and Air-conditioning Engineers
cfm	Cubic feet per minute
cfu/g	Colony forming units per gram
CO	Carbon monoxide
CO_2	Carbon dioxide
DOAS	Dedicated outdoor air system
EPA	U.S. Environmental Protection Agency
°F	Degrees Fahrenheit
FID	Flame ionization detector
HEPA	High-efficiency particulate air
HVAC	Heating, ventilating, and air-conditioning
H_2S	Hydrogen sulfide
IEQ	Indoor environmental quality
L/s	Liters per second
NAICS	North American Industry Classification System
NIOSH	National Institute for Occupational Safety and Health
OSHA	Occupational Safety and Health Administration
PID	Photionization detector
ppm	Parts per million
RH	Relative humidity
SW	Southwest
VOC	Volatile organic compound

Highlights of the NIOSH Health Hazard Evaluation

In April 2011, employees requested a health hazard evaluation to investigate concerns about indoor environmental quality at an accounting office in Florida with a history of indoor dampness, mold growth, and building-related symptoms among staff.

What NIOSH Did:

- We reviewed historical environmental reports.
- We visually assessed the office building and ventilation equipment on June 22-23, 2011.
- We took measurements of carbon dioxide, carbon monoxide, temperature, relative humidity, hydrogen sulfide, and volatile organic compounds in the air.
- We collected carpet dust samples from nine areas to analyze for microorganisms.
- We provided recommendations to the building occupants, building owner, building management, and consultants.

What NIOSH Found:

- In the interior of the building we observed:
    - ill-fitting weather stripping on exterior doors;
    - water-stained ceiling tiles, window sill, and walls;
    - raised area on cloth wallpaper from a previous water leak;
    - neutral air flow between the men's bathroom and hallway;
    - rust stains at roof lap joints in ceiling plenum; and
    - portable air cleaner units.
- On the roof, we smelled a musty odor in two air-handling units and observed dust accumulation and visible mold (confirmed by sampling) in the supply ducts inside two air-handling units.
- We observed over-sized filters in air-handling units, dusty cooling coils, build-up in drain pans, and rusty areas. We also observed condensate water from coils draining incorrectly in one air-handling unit.
- Carpet dust sampling showed heavy microbial contamination in some areas.
- Environmental reports from consultants prior to our visit reported the following findings:
    - stained ceiling tiles,
    - moisture in drywall of Room 19 window,
    - elevated relative humidity levels during some unoccupied periods,
    - water stains on wall in Hall 5 from a reported roof leak,

- visible water damage above baseboard close to exit door in Hall 11,
- wall cavity air sampling positive for fungal hyphae in Room 6 and fungi in Hall 11,
- vacuum cleaners without high-efficiency particulate air filters,
- ponding of water on a deteriorated section of the roof near a drain,
- plant growth on the roof,
- low-efficiency filters in air-handling units,
- visible mold growth confirmed by microscopic analysis in some air-handling units,
- insulation wet to touch in some air-handling units,
- no Chinese drywall.

What has been done since the NIOSH Site Visit:

- Monitored temperature and relative humidity in five areas for several days.

- Tested 13 rooms for cat, dog, cockroach, and dust mite allergens.

- Performed concrete slab testing for moisture in Rooms 2, 21, 27, and 29.

- Explored wall cavities in Halls 5 and 11 and Rooms 6, 10, and 12.

- Replaced drywall in Rooms 6 and 10 with suspect visible mold.

- Removed a vacuum that did not have a high-efficiency particulate air filter.

- Repaired window leak in Room 19.

- Increased exhaust fan air flow in the men's bathroom.

- Removed carpet and replaced with ceramic tile in Room 6 and Hall 5 and Hall 11.

- Replaced weather stripping around exterior doors at Hall 5 and Hall 11.

- Replaced asphalt landing with concrete landing and installed a wider awning at Hall 5 door.

- Waterproofed back wall and installed new French drain along the wall.

- Re-graded foundation for better drainage.

Highlights of the NIOSH Health Hazard Evalution (continued)

- Removed plants with offensive odor.
- Replaced air-handling units 1 and 4 and some fiberglass ductwork.
- Steam-cleaned carpet.
- Relocated to new building when employees continued to have building-related symptoms.

What the Next Employer/Tenant Can Do:

- Use track-off floor mats at each doorway.
- Avoid the use of chair mats; if not feasible, use perforated chair mats.
- Keep paper and boxes off the floor as much as possible.
- Clean the carpet with a high-efficiency particulate air vacuum and ensure the vacuum is well-maintained.
- Avoid the use of biocides.
- Collect carpet dust for microbial testing to determine if the carpet cleaning was successful. If there is not a significant decrease in microbes, the carpet may need to be removed.
- Avoid the use of air cleaners.
- Encourage building occupants who experience worsening, persistent, or recurrent respiratory or other health symptoms that may be associated with being in the building to see their physician.
- Implement a fragrance-free policy.

What the Building Manager/Owner Can Do:

- Perform routine maintenance of air-handling units.
- Routinely assess the building for water intrusion and damage and high relative humidity and correct these upon discovery.
- Promptly remove any future mold or moisture-damaged materials with appropriate containment.
- Do not rely upon air sampling for mold since air concentrations cannot be interpreted with respect to health risk.
- Keep a record of when and where mold or water-damaged materials are discovered and what has been done to promptly fix the problem.

NIOSH considers dampness in occupied buildings a public health problem that requires remediation. NIOSH investigators found a history of dampness and mold growth in the building and recommended remediation measures, many of which were undertaken.

What Employees Can Do:

- Inform management of any water leaks, dampness, musty or moldy odors, or ventilation problems in the building.

- See a healthcare provider if you develop or have developed recurring or worsening respiratory symptoms or other health symptoms while working in the building.

- Let your supervisor know if your healthcare provider recommends relocation to another work area to prevent exposure to mold or dampness-related contaminants that may be causing or exacerbating your symptoms.

SUMMARY

On April 15, 2011, NIOSH received an employee request regarding headaches, fatigue, weakness, fever, chills, flu-like symptoms, shortness of breath, coughing, chronic sinusitis, sore throat, burning eyes, and difficulty concentrating in a water-damaged building. In June 2011, NIOSH investigators conducted a site visit. The majority of employees reported building-related symptoms. We found evidence of water damage inside the building and mold inside supply air ducts of two air handlers. Vacuumed carpet dust samples collected during the site visit showed a high burden of culturable fungi and bacteria. We provided a number of recommendations for remediation including addressing causes of water damage and replacing contaminated carpet and ductwork. Building management replaced two rooftop air handling units and some ductwork. The carpet was steam cleaned. Some building occupants continued to have symptoms, and the accounting company relocated to another building.

Keywords: NAICS 541211 (Offices of Certified Public Accountants), indoor environmental quality, IEQ, respiratory symptoms, dampness, mold, bacteria, ventilation, HVAC, carpet

INTRODUCTION

In April 2011, the Health Hazard Evaluation (HHE) Program of the National Institute for Occupational Safety and Health (NIOSH) received a request to investigate concerns about the indoor environmental quality (IEQ) at an accounting office in Florida; at the same time we received the HHE request, we received inquiries from a Florida U.S. Senator regarding employee health concerns. The requestors reported odors and air quality problems throughout the offices. Health concerns included headaches, fatigue, weakness, fever, chills, flu-like-symptoms, shortness of breath, coughing, chronic sinusitis, dusty and metallic taste, irritated and sore throats, burning eyes, red eyes, and difficulty with thought processes.

The accounting firm resided in a two-tenant single-story building erected in 1984 near several other office buildings and strip malls. During the year prior to the firm's 2007 occupancy of the space, it was completely gutted and renovated. Their offices occupied about 7,500 square feet, or nearly two-thirds of the building, comprising 45 rooms, of which six rooms were shared with a partner financial management firm. Most were single-occupancy rooms, although there were a few open-space cubicles and two reception areas. Additionally, there were two conference rooms, bathrooms, copy rooms, three storage rooms, a file room, and a kitchen/breakroom (Figure 1). There were approximately 30 workers in the accounting office.

The building was constructed on a concrete slab and had stucco-faced concrete block exterior walls with many windows (Figures 2 and 3). Mineral-surfaced roll roofing covered the slightly sloped roof. Roof water flowed through drainpipes within the hanging ceiling plenum, exterior walls, and underground, and it emptied into a storm drainage manhole in the front parking lot (Figures 4-6). On the roof were eight heating, ventilating, and air conditioning (HVAC) air handling units (AHUs), five of which (AHU-1 through AHU-5) served the accounting office space (Figure 4). These HVAC units and the zones they served within the building are shown in Figure 1.

The floors of the main reception area and nearby hallway were wood, those of the bathroom and kitchen were tile, and the remainder of the space had low-pile carpet (Figure 7). All interior walls were drywall covered with paint, with the exception of those in two offices on the northwest side that were covered with cloth wallpaper. The hanging ceiling was composed of acoustical fiber ceiling tiles, fluorescent lighting fixtures, and the HVAC system supply and return air grilles. Inside the ceiling plenum were the corrugated metal roof deck, steel roof trusses, electrical wiring and lighting, roof drain pipes, and the HVAC supply and return air ductwork (Figures 5, 8, 9 and 10). The main duct trunk lines connected to the AHUs were made of resin-bonded fiber glass formed into rigid, rectangular boards, faced on the outside with foil (Figure 9) and a fiber glass mat on the inside airstream surface (Figure 11). From these, round flexible ducts, wrapped with foil-lined insulation, extended to the supply and return grilles mounted in the ceiling (Figure 10).

During the 2006-2007 rebuild, AHU-4 was replaced, as was all ductwork for each HVAC system. The renovation also included the closure with concrete block of an opening for a garage-type door in Room 6 used by the previous engineering firm tenant for access to surveying equipment.

METHODS

We reviewed consultant reports of several IEQ evaluations (dated March 2008 through June 2011). On June 22 and 23, 2011, we made a walk-through evaluation of the accounting office. An environmental specialist from the local county health department joined us during part of the evaluation.

We visited each room of the accounting office and those shared with the financial management firm. In nearly half of the rooms and outside, we took measurements of temperature, relative humidity, carbon dioxide (CO_2) and carbon monoxide (CO) with a Velocicalc™ multi-function ventilation meter, Model 9555-X (TSI, Inc., Shoreview, MN). Additionally, because a recent investigation had some positive findings for hydrogen sulfide (H_2S), we sampled for the compound with a GasBadge Pro™ single gas monitor for H_2S (Industrial Scientific Corp., Oakdale, PA). The health department environmental specialist simultaneously collected volatile organic compound (VOC) measurements with a TVA-1000 Toxic Vapor Analyzer™ (Thermo Environmental Instruments, Inc , Franklin, MA). This instrument has both a photoionization detector (PID) and a flame ionization detector (FID) for measurements. We used a Model DG-2 digital pressure gauge (Energy Conservatory, Minneapolis, MN) to check the air flow between the bathrooms and adjacent hallway.

As we visited each room, we looked for evidence of water damage, water incursion, visible mold, and other potential IEQ problems. We made similar inspections of the ceiling plenum. Near the floor of several rooms, we used a hand saw to cut out approximately 8 inch by 8 inch sections of drywall to look inside the wall cavities for water damage or mold growth, and then we replaced the sections and sealed them with tape (Figure 12). We inspected the exterior of the building and the roof. We opened each of the air handling units to observe the condition of the internal components and the attached supply and return ducts.

In several rooms that had previous water incursions, were adjacent to rooms that had previous water incursions, or had no previous

Methods (continued)

incursions, we collected carpet dust samples into filter socks (Model X-Cell 100, Midwest Filtration Co., Cincinnati, OH) using a L'il Hummer™ backpack vacuum (Pro-Team Inc, Boise, ID) from a 1 square meter area of the carpet for five minutes. We sealed the dust samples in plastic bags and transported them on ice to the NIOSH laboratory. At the NIOSH laboratory, we removed hair, fluff, and other large objects from the sample. We emptied each dust sample into a 15 milliliter pyrogen-free conical tube and homogenized it by rotation on a 360-degree rotary arm shaker at 65 revolutions per minute for 2 hours. We sent a 100 milligram fraction of each dust sample on ice to an environmental microbiology laboratory accredited by the American Industrial Hygiene Association (EMLab P&K, San Bruno, CA). We requested analysis of the dust samples for culturable fungi with full speciation, Gram-positive bacteria, Gram-negative bacteria, and actinomycetes.

We collected several material samples (bulk cutout, tweezed, or tape-lifted) from the inside insulated walls of two HVAC air supply ducts with suspected fungal contamination. We sent the samples in plastic bags on ice to the NIOSH laboratory. We asked for qualitative microscopic examination of the cutout, tweezed, and tape-lifted samples.

As we visited rooms, we asked the occupants about any IEQ concerns they may have had in the building.

Results

Brief summary of prior consultant reports

<u>March 2008</u>
A March 2008 consultant report noted that the southwest (SW) back door at Hall 5 had no weather stripping, the nearby indoor carpet was damp, and the adjacent ground outside needed to be re-graded below slab level; a maintenance person placed weather stripping on the door frame before the end of the consultant's inspection visit. Two ceiling tiles had small water stains. The report also noted low-efficiency filters in the rooftop AHUs. Real-time measurements collected one day throughout the building for temperature ranged from 63 degrees Fahrenheit (°F) to 71°F and for relative humidity (RH) from 33% to 48%; some of the temperatures being below the American Society of Heating,

Refrigerating, and Air-conditioning Engineers (ASHRAE) recommended acceptability range for comfort. The consultant also data-logged temperature and RH levels over seven days and found that during most of the occupied periods they were acceptable. However, he noted that during some unoccupied morning periods, many interior spaces had RH measurements above the acceptability range upper limit of 60%. He also noticed vacuum cleaners did not use high-efficiency particulate air (HEPA) filters.

July 2009

A consultant conducted an investigation into the source of odors noticed mainly near the Room 34 reception area and Hall 5. Outdoor air dampers on AHU-2, AHU-3, and AHU-5 were found to be closed. He noted ponding of water on a deteriorated section of roof material near a drain used for AHU-1 and AHU-2 condensate drainage, and he observed a plant growing in the roof material. He reported that the roof was likely breached, based on water staining observed on the underside of the roof assembly near the drain for AHU-1 and AHU-2. Finding no indoor odor sources, the consultant suspected outdoor sources.

June 2010

A consultant in June 2010 noticed no odors during his investigation. He reported moisture in the drywall at the bottom right corner of the window in Room 19 and recommended removal of a one foot section of the damaged window sill. He also noted water stains on the interior side of the roof assembly without ceiling tile staining. Low-efficiency filters were in some of the air handlers. Indoor RH measurements were 58%–61%. Concentrations of fungal spores found in indoor air were equal to or lower than outdoors. The consultant also reported visible mold growth (confirmed by microscopic analysis) in some of the air handlers, as well as some with insulation that was wet to the touch. Surface samples taken from ducts at the AHUs identified a large quantity of mold spores, hyphae, and black opaque particulates. He also found similar black opaque particulates on some horizontal surfaces inside the building and noted they were not consistent with typical indoor dust but probably came from outside, and they may have been contributing to the odor and symptoms described by the employees.

October 2010

A consultant using a moisture meter reported no current moisture on tested materials in the building. He found water stains on a Hall 5 interior wall (shared with Room 3) from a reported roof leak. He also reported visible water damage (paint peeling) above the baseboard close to the exit door on the Hall 11 west wall shared with Room 10. He performed wall cavity spore trap sampling in the Hall 11 water-damaged wall (shared with Room 10) and in the exterior walls of Hall 5 and Room 6. In Hall 11, he found *Aspergillus/Pencillium*-like, Basidiospores, *Cladosporium*, and *Stachybotrys* spores. He was unable to evaluate the east wall (shared with office 12) because of furniture along that wall. In the Room 6 wall, the consultant found hyphal fragments, while the wall cavity sampling was negative in Hall 5. He recommended removal of the damaged section of the west wall (shared with Room 10) in Hall 11 for inspection and repair. He also reported that the adjacent exterior door needed to be properly sealed.

October-November 2010 (picture documentation)
In October, the building manager inspected the wall between Hall 5 and Room 3. We were told by building occupants that a plugged AHU-1 condensate drain caused water to leak into the wall. The building manager replaced the baseboard in room 3 along the wall shared with Hall 5, and suspect mold was found (Figure 13). The damaged section of the drywall was removed (Figure 14), and the baseboard was replaced. In November, a large section hole was cut near the base of the Hall 5 wall shared with Room 3. No visible mold was found (Figures 15-18).

April 2011
During an Occupational Safety and Health Administration (OSHA) inspection on April 4, 2011, the inspector measured 8-hour time-weighted average H_2S concentrations of 0.26, 0.95, and 0.33 parts per million (ppm), respectively, outside, and inside on personal samplers in Room 6 and in a cubicle across the hall from Room 3. Two other samples from Rooms 12 and 25 did not have any H_2S detected.

June 2011
An engineering consultant evaluated the building in May 2011 to determine if it contained Chinese drywall. Based on visual observations of copper throughout the building and laboratory testing of drywall samples, they concluded there was no Chinese drywall in the building.

NIOSH June 2011 site visit

Walkthrough evaluation

During our walk-through of the building on June 22, the average inside temperature around 3:00 p.m. was 72°F, and the RH was 56%, while it was 88°F with an RH of 65% outside (Table 1). An average of 642 ppm CO_2 was found inside, while it was 416 ppm outside. A few trace measurements of CO were obtained in some rooms on the northwest side of the building; CO was not detected elsewhere. H_2S was not detected anywhere, inside or outside, including on the roof directly above sewer vents. The vapor analyzer measured an average of 0.1 ppm VOCs inside and 0.2 ppm outside with its PID. Simultaneously, its FID measured an average of 1 5 ppm inside and 2.0 ppm outside. We smelled perfumes and colognes in multiple rooms.

We observed stained ceiling tiles in Room 23 and the adjoining hallway (both at the shared wall) and Rooms 28, 32, and 37. Investigation of the sources indicated that the stains in Room 23 (Figures 19 and 20) and the adjoining hall were likely associated with the penetration area of an AHU-5 duct through the roof. The Room 37 stain was under a roof drain penetration (Figures 21 and 22). A small nail-sized hole in the metal roof panel was located directly above the stained tile in Room 28, and the stain in Room 32 was under a roof lap joint.

In Room 3, on the wall shared with Hall 5, there was a raised area of the cloth wall paper from the ceiling down that was likely from the water leak that had previously occurred (Figure 23). In Room 19, we observed water stains and blistering paint on the window sill (Figures 24 and 25). By the middle exterior door in Hall 11, we observed vertical water drip marks on the bottom half of the wall shared with Room 10 (Figure 26) that may have come from rain water falling from clothes and/or umbrellas as people enter.

In the ceiling plenum, we saw the cement-like roof insulation material, noted in previous reports that appeared to have oozed out from some roof lap joints during construction (Figures 27 and 28). Some of the roof lap joints had rusty stains, but none appeared to be wet (Figures 29 and 30). The HVAC flexible ducts appeared to be tightly fitted to main trunk lines and supply and return grilles; however, some of the flexible ducts probably had reduced air flow from being crimped by wire hangers (Figure 10). A coating of fine dust was seen on most of the trusses, ducts, and pipes in the plenum (Figures 5, 8, 9, 10, 27, 29, and 30). Because it was not also seen on the ceiling supports and tiles, and the HVAC system is fully ducted, it was likely construction dust.

We found the men's bathroom to be neutrally pressurized in relation to the hallway. The women's bathroom exhaust fan was able to keep it correctly negatively pressurized, thus preventing odors from escaping from the room.

In Room 6, we observed a portable HEPA air cleaner unit. Room 28 and the bathrooms had portable ultraviolet air cleaners.

We observed three custodial staff vacuuming carpets after business hours. Two vacuums had HEPA filters, and one did not.

We noted ill-fitting weather stripping around both back doors (Figures 31 and 32). Canvas awnings hung above each door, to the width of the door at Hall 5 (Figure 33a) and to the extent of the adjoining windows at the door at Hall 11 (Figure 34). Building occupants reported that the canvas awnings had been installed within the prior year.

On the roof, we observed no puddling of water from the rainfall just prior to our roof inspection, and the roofing material appeared to be in good condition. We found over-sized high-efficiency filters (Figure 35) in AHU-1, AHU-2, AHU-3, and AHU-5, causing gaps which allowed air to bypass the filters. In AHU-4, condensate water from the coils was found in the filter housing base and dripping into the outside air and return air mixing plenum rather than draining correctly to the drain (Figure 36). The bottom of the filter was wet. We smelled a musty odor and observed dust accumulation and suspect mold growth in AHU-1 (Figure 37) and AHU-4 (Figures 38 and 39a) supply ducts immediately after the fans. Other supply ducts and all return ducts viewed inside the AHUs had only minimal dust accumulation (Figure 39b). We observed dusty cooling coils (Figures 40 and 41), build-up in drain pans, and rusty areas in AHUs (Figures 42-44).

Building occupants reported episodes of water intrusion that resulted in wet carpet. They reported a history of frequent water leaks at the middle back door (Hall 11) and SW back door (Hall 5) which improved after awnings were installed above the doors (Figures 33a and 34). They also reported that water had wet the carpet in the storage room (by Room 25) from a leak behind the back wall of the storage room, and when the water leaked from AHU-1, the carpet near the wall shared by Hall 5 and Room 3 became wet. The wet carpet in all the above instances was reported to have been left to air dry, with no aggressive drying.

We spoke with all the occupants of the accounting office and the majority reported building-related symptoms. Many reported one or more mucous membrane type symptoms including dry, itchy, or burning eyes; nasal dryness; dry throat; hoarseness; sneezing; or sinus problems. Others reported symptoms including coughing, fatigue, and rashes. A number of occupants reported frequently smelling odors described in various ways, including burning rubber smell, mildew smell, moldy smell, musty smell, wet-dog smell, sewage smell, sulfur smell, and rotten egg smell.

Wall cavity exploration

We did not find evidence of moisture, water damage, mold growth, or odor in any of the wall cavities evaluated. We, and the consultants in 2010, were unable to check inside the east wall in Hall 11 due to large shelving units on either side of the wall. We were also unable to evaluate the wall in Room 6 shared with Hall 5 because of large file cabinets on both sides of the wall.

Carpet dust samples

Table 2 summarizes numbers and species of fungi and bacteria cultured from the carpet dust samples. Total fungi ranged from 12,000 colony forming units per gram (cfu/g) in Room 2 to 2,500,000 cfu/g by the SW back door (Hall 5). Total bacteria ranged from 25,000 cfu/g in Room 31 to 100,000,000 cfu/g by the SW back door. *Bacillus*, a Gram-positive bacteria, was highest by the SW back door in Hall 5 and the middle back door in Hall 11. Thermophilic actinomycetes were detected in Halls 5 and 11, Rooms 2, 6, 29, and 31, and in the storage area by Room 25.

HVAC samples

Cladosporium was cultured on both bulk cutout samples (Table 3) taken from supply ducts above the ceiling in Room 3 (HVAC-1) and the hallway near Room 12 (HVAC-4). The microscopic examination report (Table 4) indicated mold growth (indicated by hyphae) on those samples, as well as samples obtained from the same supply ducts at the rooftop AHUs.

Closing meeting at end of site visit

During the closing meeting, we recommended the following:

1. Replace fiberglass ducts for HVAC systems 1 and 4.

2. Replace weather stripping on Hall 5 and Hall 11 back doors.

3. Increase the air flow in the men's bathroom to put the bathroom under negative pressure in relation to the hallway.

4. Evaluate the window in Room 19 for water leaks and fix any leaks.

5. Evaluate source of leaks for the stained ceiling tiles.

6. Repair water leaks to prevent further water entry into the building.

7. Remove or clean mold and moisture-damaged materials with appropriate containment to minimize exposure of building occupants.

8. During and after heavy rains, walk through the building to check for water incursion.

9. Remove filtration/sanitizer devices in the bathrooms.

10. Implement a fragrance-free policy.

Update since Site Visit

Below is a brief summary of follow-up after our site visit in June 2011.

<u>July 2011</u>

We shared the carpet dust and bulk material sampling results with the stakeholders. We recommended that the carpet be replaced with hard floors in Halls 5 and 11 partly because these are high traffic areas. In the other rooms, we recommended that the carpet be replaced with new carpet or hard floors. We suggested for rooms that were not tested that carpet dust sampling be performed, or the carpet be replaced similarly with the other rooms. We also suggested that concrete slab testing for moisture content would help in the selection of appropriate flooring. If new carpet would be installed, we recommended low VOC emitting carpet and adhesives be used. We recommended that carpet biocides not be used but that carpets be routinely HEPA vacuumed. We recommended that the non-HEPA vacuum that we observed during our visit be removed from the building and that the HEPA-vacuums be properly maintained. We also recommended track-off

RESULTS (CONTINUED)

floor mats at all entries.

August 2011

We had a teleconference with industrial hygiene consultants hired by the building owner/management company; we reviewed our findings and recommendations and provided our carpet sampling protocol. In a letter from the building management company, dated August 8, 2011, it was reported that the window leak in Room 19 was repaired.

We provided our written interim findings and recommendations to the stakeholders. We recommended the following:

HVAC
1. Ensure proper maintenance of HVAC units.
2. Replace incorrectly sized HVAC filters.
3. Develop a regular maintenance schedule.
4. Replace fiberglass ductwork for AHU-1 and AHU-4, preferably with metal ductwork with external insulation.
5. Replace or test fiberglass ducts for AHU-2, AHU-3, and AHU-5 for mold contamination.
6. Consult with ventilation engineers.

Carpet
1. Install track-off floor mats at exterior doors.
2. Routinely vacuum carpet with HEPA vacuum.
3. Conduct additional slab moisture testing (e g , perimeter of slab, Hall 5, Hall 11, Room 6, Room 12) to determine if there are any concrete slab moisture issues and to help in selecting appropriate flooring.
4. Replace contaminated carpet (under conditions of containment and isolation) by exterior doorways (Hall 5 and Hall 11) with hard floors.
5. Replace carpet (under conditions of containment and isolation) in the other areas sampled (areas 2, 6, 11, 12, storage room by room 25, 29, 31) with new carpet or hard floors taking into account slab moisture results.
6. Replace carpet in other rooms not sampled by NIOSH, or conduct carpet sampling in these rooms.
7. HEPA vacuum upholstered furniture.

We had been informed by an the industrial hygiene consultant that the building owner planned to replace the carpet with hard floors by the middle back door (Hall 11) and SW back door (Hall 5). In the other areas, the industrial hygiene consultant informed us that the owner planned to clean the carpets and then resample the carpets. We recommended against a water cleaning method because water-loving fungi/yeast and bacteria were present in the carpet. If the cleaning method would involve water such as hot water extraction, we noted that drying would be very important and would likely require large fans and possibly running the ventilation system during the night hours to ensure continuous airflow. Additionally, the building occupants would need advance notice so that they could box up their belongings before the cleaning. Also furniture would need to be removed from the rooms before the cleaning. We did not recommend the use of carpet biocides as a routine practice. However, if biocides were used during the cleaning process, we recommended that the manufacturer's recommendations for dilution, application, and worker protection (skin and respiratory protection) be followed. We also noted that with sufficient access to water, microorganisms in carpet can proliferate so it would be important that the sources of moisture be remediated to prevent recontamination of new or cleaned carpet. If the carpet continued to be contaminated after cleaning, we recommended it be replaced.

Roof
1. Check for any roof leaks during and after heavy rains. This would include removing ceiling tiles to check the underside of the roof.

2. Repair any roof leaks found.

Ceiling
1. Determine water source for ceiling stains and repair any defects leading to water intrusion or leaks.

2. Replace stained ceiling tiles.

Wall
1. Remove a section of the west wall (shared with Room 10) by the middle back door (Hall 11) to inspect for water damage or mold growth. We recommended removal of a section from the exterior door frame out at least 5 linear feet and at least 2 feet up from the floor. We recommended taking pictures of the findings, and if there was water damage or mold growth, remove the affected areas and repair the wall (using proper containment and isolation methods).

2. In Room 12, remove a section of the west wall (shared with Hall 11) to inspect for water damage or mold growth. We recommended removal of a section from the back (south) wall out at least 5 linear feet and at least 2 feet up from the floor and a similarly-sized section of the back wall immediately adjacent to the west wall (shared with Hall 11). We again recommended taking pictures of the findings, and if there was water damage or mold growth, remove the affected areas and repair the wall (using proper containment and isolation methods).

3. In Room 6, remove a section of the west wall (shared with area 5) to inspect for water damage or mold growth. We recommended removal of a section from the back (south) wall out at least 5 linear feet and at least 2 feet up from the floor and a similarly-sized section of the back wall immediately adjacent to the west wall (shared with Hall 5). As noted above we recommended taking pictures of the finding, and if there was water damage or mold growth, remove the affected areas and repair the wall (using proper containment and isolation methods).

Other

1. Replace weather stripping around SW back door and middle back door.

2. Fix exhaust fan in men's bathroom so it was under negative pressure in relation to the corridor.

3. Determine the source of the water stain on the window sill in Room 19 and repair.

4. Remove filtration/sanitizer devices in bathrooms.

5. Implement a fragrance-free policy.

6. Walkthrough the building during and after heavy rains to check for leaks. Keep records of damp areas and repairs.

7. During remediation, use proper isolation and containment methods to minimize exposures to remediation workers, building occupants, and unaffected sections of the building.

8. Communicate remediation plans and timeline with the building occupants in advance.

Also in August 2011, an HVAC contractor for the building owner placed temperature and RH data-logging monitors in several locations for five days. In the front reception area, Cubicle 16, and Room 29, the temperature ranged from approximately 70°F to 75°F, and the RH ranged from approximately 48% to 56%. In the work area across from Room 2, the temperature ranged from approximately 70°F to 74°F, and the RH ranged from approximately 48% to 62%. In Room 2, the temperature ranged from approximately 66°F to 74°F, and the RH ranged from 54% to 64%.

Later in August 2011, an industrial hygiene consultant took room air temperature and RH measurements at the end of concrete slab moisture testing in Rooms 2, 21, 27, and 29. At around 6:00 p.m., the temperatures in the rooms ranged from 68.9°F to 73 5°F, and the RH ranged from 44% to 53%. The reported relative humidity of the concrete ranged from 48.5% to 59%.

The industrial hygiene consultant in a letter dated August 15, 2011 reported the exhaust fan air flow for the men's bathroom was increased. Carpet was removed, and replaced with ceramic tile in Room 6, Hall 5, and Hall 11.

September 2011
We provided requested information to building occupants about how to conduct wall cavity inspections.

The property management company had replaced the weather stripping around the exterior doors. At the Hall 5 door, the asphalt landing was replaced with a concrete landing and a wider awning was installed (Figure 33b). The southwest wall (back wall with two exterior doors) was waterproofed and a new French drain was installed along the wall. Additionally, some plants that had an offensive odor were removed and the foundation was re-graded for better drainage.

October - November 2011
An industrial hygiene consultant letter dated October 10, 2011 reported remediation activities at the office building up to that date. The document reported that during their wall cavity exploration, suspect visible mold was found in Rooms 6 and 10. In Room 6, water stains, rust on the floor plates, and leaves were observed in the back wall cavity; suspect mold was observed on an approximately one foot long section of the bottom edge of the drywall. The document stated the drywall was replaced. In Room 10, suspect mold was reported on drywall in the southeast corner (back left corner as enter the room). This drywall was

also removed and replaced. The letter indicated the wall cavities were clean, and no visible mold or water stains were found in the Room 6 northwest wall shared with Hall 5, Room 10 southwest wall (exterior back wall), Room 12 northwest wall shared with Hall 11, and Room 12 southwest wall (exterior back wall). The letter also mentioned that a new French drain had been installed along the southwest wall (rear) and that the wall had been waterproofed ("stripped down to block, sealed, and coated with new waterproof stucco"). The industrial hygiene consultant emailed NIOSH multiple pictures of the wall cavity exploration.

We recommended they evaluate the two wall cavities in Room 4, specifically, in the back wall and the wall shared with Hall 5. In a letter dated December 2, 2001, the industrial hygiene consultant felt that it was not necessary and noted that the backside of Room 4's wall shared with Hall 5 was clean, and there was no evidence of water or mold damage. The letter reported that the building management company had removed and replaced approximately 175 square feet of drywall; less than one square foot had visible mold. We were also informed by the industrial hygiene consultant during a teleconference that no water damage was noted on the exterior of the southwest wall.

On October 24, 2011, the industrial hygiene consultant collected dust in 13 rooms (1, 2, 4, 10, 12, 17, 20, 27, 29, 31, 34, 35, and copy room) to test for allergens. The collection method was not described, but we assume it was settled dust (not airborne dust). The samples were analyzed using ELISA methodology for cat (Fel d1), dog (Can f1), cockroach (Bla g1), and dust mite (Der f1 and Der p1) allergens. The samples were below the limit of detection for dust mite (<0.39 microgram (μg)/gram) and cockroach (<1.6 units/gram) allergens. All 13 rooms had detectable levels of cat allergen that ranged from 0.35 μg/gram +/- 0.036 in Room 2 to 4.23 μg/gram +\-0.44 in Room 12. Six rooms were below 1 μg /gram; three rooms were between 1-2 μg /gram, and three were between 2-3 μg /gram. Ten rooms had detectable levels of dog allergen that ranged from 0.62 μg/gram +/-0.13 in Room 17 to greater than 25 μg/gram in Room 20. Nine of the 10 measurements from rooms with dog allergen were ≤ 2.5 μg /gram. Rooms 1, 2, and 10 had no detectable levels of dog allergen.

We received a carpet cleaning protocol dated October 28, 2011 from the industrial hygiene consultant. It included the optional use of tannic acid or borate solution. If carpet cleaning was attempted, we recommended dry steam cleaning which uses a high temperature, low moisture vapor, usually below 6% of water content. During our carpet dust sampling for bacteria and fungi in June 2011, we found water-loving fungi/yeast and Gram-negative and Gram-positive bacteria. We thought that adding water to the carpet by using a "wet" method was not a good idea. We did not recommend using borate or tannic acid during the cleaning process. Before the carpet cleaning, we recommended HEPA-vacuuming each room before and after removal of office contents to help reduce the suspension of carpet dust and limit contamination. We also recommended sufficient drying of the carpet after the cleaning process and HEPA-vacuuming the rooms before replacing the office contents. Additionally, we recommended carpet dust sampling after the carpet cleaning to determine if the cleaning had been successful. The results could be compared with the NIOSH carpet dust sample results collected in June 2011.

A letter dated October 27, 2011 from the engineering consultant recommended adding exhaust fans in the copy rooms, enhanced housekeeping, storing boxes off the floor, daily HEPA-vacuuming, using perforated floor mats, and replacement of AHU-1 and AHU-4. We agreed with these recommendations. We also recommended monitoring the concrete slab in a few more areas to look for moisture intrusion rates.

We thought the planned ventilation renovations seemed reasonable including the replacement of air handling units AHU-1 and AHU-4. We also thought the inclusion of a dedicated outdoor air system (DOAS), mentioned in a report dated October 27, would alleviate the outside air cooling load (especially the latent heat that is responsible for condensation and possibly microbial growth) from the other AHUs. That system, if designed properly, should alleviate most (if not all) condensation on the coils in the other AHUs and allow them to provide better temperature/humidity control in the occupied spaces. Also, a properly designed DOAS would ensure ASHRAE-recommended levels of fresh, outside air to the building occupants at all times throughout the year without significantly affecting the operating parameters of the other AHUs. A letter from the engineering consultant dated November 10, 2011 did not mention the DOAS in the context of the replacement of AHU-1 and AHU-4. We thought the recommended replacement of AHU-1 with a smaller 4 ton unit would allow additional runtime as stated in the letter. We also liked the idea of a 2-stage unit for AHU-4 if the DOAS was not added. In a letter dated November 1,

2011 from the engineering consultant, the engineer recommended removal of AHU-1 main ductwork through the first two sections of horizontal ductwork off the unit and that remaining ductwork would be removed until visually found to be clean as verified by the engineer or his representative. For AHU-4, the engineer consultant also recommended that the main ductwork be removed and replaced throughout the main duct run.

In November 2011, AHU-4 was changed to a 2-stage unit to increase the time that active cooling was occurring and to increase the ventilation that was brought into the area served by the unit. AHU-1 was downsized to better match the load of the area served. Some of the fiberglass ductwork was also replaced.

December 2011
We provided the building occupants with a requested carpet removal protocol for the accounting office.

We had a teleconference with industrial hygiene and engineering consultants hired by the building owner/manager. There was a question about the condensate drainage for AHU-4. This was evaluated about a week later by an employee for the engineering company. The condensate drain was reported to drain properly. The AHU-4 was also reported to be properly trapped, and the inside of the unit and ductwork connected to the unit were reported to be clean and dry. The ceiling tiles below the unit were reported to be clean and unstained.

February/March 2012
A building occupant reported finding two to three silver dollar size spots resembling mold on the carpet under a chair mat in Room 13.

In late February or early March, the carpet in the accounting office was steam cleaned.

November 2012
A building occupant informed us that some building occupants continued to have symptoms, and the accounting company would be relocating to another building.

December 2012
The accounting company relocated to another building. The remaining carpet had not been tested (carpet dust) or replaced prior to moving.

DISCUSSION

Occupants of this building had a several-year history of building-related symptoms, which was reflected in recurrent complaints to the building management company and several consultant reports from 2008 until the time of the NIOSH survey in June 2011. Workers reported water damage reflected in stained ceilings and walls. Consultants had findings reflecting water damage, also including stained ceiling tiles as well as visible mold and wall cavity sampling identifying *Stachybotrys*, a water-loving fungus [Hung et al. 2005] that is not normally present on building materials [Prezant et al. 2008] and reflects wet indoor conditions. Nonetheless, confusion about the nature and source of odors resulted in exploring other explanations such as hydrogen sulfide and Chinese drywall, rather than remediating dampness or accepting that indoor dampness was an adequate cause for occupants' indoor environmental quality complaints. There is growing epidemiological evidence of associations between respiratory health effects and microbial contaminants derived from mold and bacteria, allergens from dust mites and cockroaches, and chemical agents released from wetted building materials and furnishings [IOM 2004; WHO 2009].

Symptoms

The occupants reported symptoms consistent with damp indoor environments. In 2004, the Institute of Medicine (IOM) of the National Academies published an extensive review of past scientific studies on the health effects of damp buildings [IOM 2004]. In 2009, the World Health Organization (WHO) published guidelines for dampness and mold based on an updated review [WHO 2009]. The WHO report points out that (1) *clinical evidence* is *sufficient* to conclude that exposure to mold and other dampness-related microbial agents in the indoor environment increases the risk of hypersensitivity pneumonitis, chronic rhinosinusitis, and allergic fungal sinusitis; (2) *epidemiological evidence is sufficient* to conclude that occupants of damp or moldy buildings are at increased risk of respiratory symptoms (specifically upper respiratory tract symptoms, cough, wheeze, and shortness of breath), respiratory infections, asthma development, current asthma, and asthma exacerbation; and (3) *epidemiological evidence suggests* that occupants of damp or moldy buildings are also at increased risk of bronchitis and allergic rhinitis. Importantly, the WHO guidelines note that although allergy and atopy (genetic tendency to develop allergic diseases such as atopic dermatitis, hay fever, and asthma) increases susceptibility to dampness-related health effects, such health effects are also found in non-atopic building occupants. Additional evidence from a more recent epidemiologic review reported that bronchitis, shortness of breath, and eczema should be added to the list of health outcomes with sufficient evidence of an association to dampness and dampness-related agents [Mendell et al. 2011]. Vocal-cord dysfunction has also been reported in workers in water-damaged buildings [Cummings et al. 2013].

Microbial contamination – carpet and ventilation supply ducts

Bacteria, fungi, actinomycetes, and non-tuberculous mycobacteria have been associated with damp indoor environments. In this building, bacteria, fungi, and actinomycetes were identified in the carpet dust samples and in bulk material collected from inside the ventilation insulation board supply ducts. The carpet dust samples we collected had Gram-negative bacteria, which suggest indoor sources of dampness [Burge 1994], and many fungi that grow in environments with high or moderate water activity (e.g., yeasts, *Phoma* spp, *Alternaria alternata, Aspergus niger, Aspergillus ochraceus, Cladosporium cladosporioides, Penicillium brevicompactum*) [Hung et al. 2005]. The spectrum of fungal species identified indicate that the carpet likely experienced chronic wet conditions in the past or alternating cycles of wet and dry conditions. Currently, there are no standards for what level or what species of molds constitute a health risk. For example, all molds have the potential to be allergenic, but little knowledge exits on the antigens or allergens found in the vast majority of molds. An OSHA technical manual [1999] reports contamination indicators of 1,000,000 fungi per gram of dust or material; however, this is not based on health risk. Dr. Burge, EMLab P&K's Director of Aerobiology, also reported unusual levels of microorganisms in dust samples [Burge 2010]. However, there are no accepted quantitation levels for health effects for microorganisms in carpet dust.

Thermophilic actinomycetes were detected in all the carpet and the bulk material collected from inside the ventilation insulation board supply ducts, which likely resulted in the circulation of the microbes throughout the building. Thermophilic actinomycetes are bacteria that thrive at higher temperatures and cause hypersensitivity pneumonitis (also referred to as extrinsic allergic alveolitis) [Eduard 2009]. Hypersensitivity pneumonitis is an immunologically-mediated, granulomatous lung disease caused by repeated inhalation and sensitization to various organic agents including microbial agents [Girard et al. 2004].

In this building, the carpet was replaced with hard flooring in one office and at the door entries. The rest of the carpet was steam cleaned. The steam cleaned carpet was not re-sampled (carpet dust) to determine if the cleaning had effectively removed the microbial contamination. If the carpet is still contaminated with microbes, this may have accounted for some of the continued symptoms in building occupants.

The contaminated fiberglass ducts were reported to have been replaced with fiberglass ducts. Because fiberglass ducts can have a rough surface, they often make an excellent trap for dust. A lot of dust is organic dust, which will often grow mold and bacteria with moisture. Fiberglass insulation that has mold growth must be replaced because it cannot be cleaned. Smooth metal interior ductwork is often a better alternative. It will be important to properly maintain the HVAC units to prevent future contamination.

We do not recommend the use of biocides on carpet or in the HVAC system. The growth of mold and bacteria in indoor environments is due to excess moisture; thus, application of biocide as a protective action is unnecessary if moisture is properly controlled. Biocides should not be applied in an occupied building or in an operating HVAC system [Sesline et al. 1994]. Any biocide use on carpet or in HVAC systems or ductwork, even EPA-approved biocides, should be minimized, carefully monitored in terms of occupant health and air quality, and guided by professional judgment [Prezant et al. 2008].

Indoor relative humidity and temperature

Controlling indoor relative humidity is also an important factor to prevent microbial growth in the ventilation ducts and carpet. During our visit, indoor relative humidity measurements were within normal range; however, some RH measurements were on the high end of normal. This was also observed in 2008 when a consultant recorded indoor relative humidity levels above 60%, mainly during unoccupied periods in the early morning hours, and in August 2011 when a consultant measured peak indoor humidity readings of 62% and 64%. In the United States, ASHRAE recommends that indoor RH be maintained at or below 65% [ANSI/ASHRAE 2010A]. The U.S. Environmental Protection

Discussion (continued)

Agency (EPA) recommends maintaining indoor RH between 30%–50% because excessive humidity can promote the excessive growth of microorganisms [EPA 2008]. During our evaluation, the HVAC systems were running during occupied hours and turned off at night. While turning the system off may seem more economic, it also increases demand on the system when it is turned back on to reach desired temperature set-points. It can also create issues with humidity and condensation if temperatures indoors become warm during the "off" periods. This is particularly true in areas with warmer climates such as Florida.

Assuming slow air movement and 50% RH, the operative temperatures recommended by ASHRAE range from 68.5°F–76°F in the winter, and from 75.5°F–80 5°F in the summer (see table below). The difference between the two is largely due to seasonal clothing selection [ANSI/ASHRAE 2010A]. During our summertime visit, the indoor temperature averaged 72°F, a few degrees below the lower range recommended by ASHRAE. However, if building occupants feel comfortable at that temperature, then there is no real reason for concern as long as RH levels remain controlled.

Relative Humidity	Winter Temperatures[1]	Summer Temperatures[1]
30%[2]	69.5–77.0 °F	75.5–81.5 °F
40%	69.0–76.5 °F	75.5–81.0 °F
50%[3]	68.5–76.0 °F	75.0–80.5 °F

[1] Applies to occupants wearing typical summer and winter clothing, with a sedentary to light activity level.
[2] Humidity levels below 30% may cause irritated mucus membranes, dry eyes, and sinus discomfort.
[3] EPA recommends maintaining indoor RH below 60% and ideally in a range from 30%–50% to prevent mold growth.

Ventilation

During our visit, the office building had adequate ventilation during the day based on carbon dioxide (CO_2) levels. ASHRAE notes in an appendix to standard American National Standards Institute (ANSI)/ASHRAE 62.1-2010: *Ventilation for Acceptable Indoor Air Quality* that indoor CO_2 concentrations no greater than 700 ppm above outdoor CO_2 concentrations will satisfy a substantial majority (about 80%) of visitors with regard to odor from sedentary building occupants (body odor) [ANSI/ASHRAE,

2010B]. This would typically correspond to indoor concentrations below 1200 ppm since outdoor CO_2 concentrations usually range between 375 to 500 ppm. Elevated CO_2 concentrations in a building suggest that other indoor contaminants may also be increased and that the amount of outdoor air introduced into the ventilated space to dilute those pollutants may need to be increased. CO_2 is not an effective indicator of ventilation adequacy if the ventilated area is not occupied at its usual occupant density at the time the CO_2 is measured.

ASHRAE guidelines provide specific details on ventilation for acceptable indoor environmental quality. ANSI/ASHRAE Standard 62.1-2010: *Ventilation for Acceptable Indoor Air Quality* specifies "minimum ventilation rates and other measures intended to provide indoor air quality that is acceptable to human occupants and that minimize adverse health effects"[ANSI/ASHRAE 2010B]. Generally, the standard recommends outdoor air supply rates to indoor occupied spaces that take into account people-related sources as well as building-related sources. For office spaces, conference rooms, and reception areas, 2.5 liters per second per person (L/s·person) (5 cubic feet per minute [cfm] of outside air per person [cfm/person]) is recommended for people-related sources, and an additional 0.3 liters per second per square meter (L/s·m²) (0.06 cfm per square foot [cfm/ft²]) of occupied space is recommended to account for building-related sources. For spaces where airborne contaminants and odors are prevalent, the standard offers minimum exhaust rates from the space. For copy and printing rooms, the standard recommends an exhaust rate of at least 2.5 L/s·m² (0.5 cfm/ft²) directly outdoors. The makeup air for this exhaust air can consist of any combination of outdoor air, recirculated air, or air transferred from adjacent spaces. When normal dilution ventilation does not reduce occupant exposures to emissions from office equipment to acceptable levels, some form of local exhaust ventilation must be considered to remove the contaminant from the source before it can be spread throughout the occupied space. However, little scientific research has been done to develop and/or test the performance of local exhaust systems for typical office equipment.

Portable Air Cleaners

We observed a portable HEPA air cleaner unit and ultraviolet air cleaners during our site visit. HEPA units are made to remove particles from the air, which could include some mists. Ultraviolet air cleaners kills living organisms. Portable air cleaners should not be necessary if there is appropriate ventilation and no issues with indoor dampness. Portable air cleaners that produce ozone can cause adverse respiratory health effects and should be avoided [EPA 2009 and 2013].

Cat and Dog Allergens

In 2011, cat (Fel d 1) and/or dog (Can f 1) allergens were identified in dust samples collected by an industrial hygiene consultant at the accounting office. The consultant found cat allergen in more rooms than dog allergen which is common. Cat allergens are ubiquitous, being found in homes with and without cats and in many schools and office buildings; the levels of allergens in office buildings and schools are generally lower than residential exposures [Cox-Ganser et al. 2010]. Cat and dog allergens are transported on the clothing of people (such as employees and visitors) who have household pets to pet-free areas such as workplaces [Perfetti et al. 2004]. Multiple studies have shown dog and cat allergens on carpet and often much higher levels on upholstered chairs in public places and indoor workplaces [Custovic et al. 1996, 1998; Perfetti et al. 2004]. These passively transferred allergens can become airborne and cause respiratory symptoms in individuals allergic to cats or dogs. In general, the lower the level of allergen in the environment, the lower the risk of allergic symptoms.

Fragrances

During our visit, we smelled perfumes and colognes in multiple rooms. No building occupants complained about the perfume or cologne scent. Several hundred different chemicals are used to make fragrances, many with little available health data. Fragranced products have been implicated in causing dermatologic problems [Buckley et al. 2002] and inducing or worsening respiratory problems [Bridges 2002] including asthma [Baldwin et al 1999; Kumar et al. 1995; Caress and Steinemann 2009] and vocal cord dysfunction [Hoy et al. 2010]. Fragranced products are reported to trigger symptoms in individuals with asthma [Baldwin et al 1999; Kumar et al. 1995; Caress and Steinemann 2009], hay fever [Baldwin et al 1999], and migraines [Kelman 2004 and 2007], even when the individuals are not "allergic" to fragrance ingredients. In one study, investigators collected data through telephone interviews from two geographically weighted, random samples in the continental U.S. in surveys during 2002-2003 (1,057 participants) and 2005-2006 (1,058 participants). Results aggregated from both surveys found that 30.5% of the general population reported scented products irritating and 19% reported adverse health effects such as headaches and breathing problems [Caress and Steinemann 2009].

We recommended that the management at the accounting office implement a fragance-free policy. Many employers have established fragrance-free policies in their workplaces to protect their workers who are symptomatic when exposed to products that contain fragrances. These policies generally prohibit the use of the following types of scented products anywhere in their buildings: perfumes and colognes, deodorants, hairsprays, lotions and creams, potpourri, air fresheners, candles, scented soaps and cleaning chemicals, and any other fragrance-containing products. In addition, use of soaps and cleaning products by janitorial staff can be limited to products that are fragrance-free or emit only low levels of VOCs. Workers can also be encouraged to be as fragrance-free as possible upon arrival at the buildings, including not only the personal care products used on their skin, but also by avoiding use of scented detergents and fabric softeners on clothes worn to the building.

Health Outcomes Following Remediation

Numerous studies have documented health outcomes following remediation of water-damaged buildings. In some buildings, remediation has been followed by decreases in respiratory symptoms reported by occupants [Jarvis and Morey 2001; Haverinen-Shaughnessy et al. 2004; Meklin et al. 2005; Kercsmar et al. 2006; Lignell et al. 2007; Haverinen-Shaughnessy et al. 2008] and no new cases of respiratory illness [Jarvis and Morey 2001]. In other buildings, remediation has not resulted in improved health outcomes. Incomplete remediation is one possible explanation [Ebbehoj et al. 2002; Patovirta et al. 2004; Meklin et al. 2005; Haverinen-Shaughnessy et al. 2008; Iossifova 2011]. Yet there is also evidence that remediation may be effective in terms of preventing new illness, but not eliminating symptoms in previously affected occupants [Haverinen-Shaughnessy et al. 2004]. For some employees, an individualized management plan (such as assigning an affected employee to a different work location, perhaps at home or a remote site) is required, depending upon medical findings and recommendations of the individual's physician.

CONCLUSIONS

The building-related symptoms experienced by many employees in this building are consistent with diverse exposures found in damp indoor buildings. There was evidence for dampness in occupant observations, historical consultant reports, NIOSH findings of unusual high levels of microrganisms requiring damp indoor environments in carpet dust, HVAC contamination, and interior water stains on ceiling tiles and walls. Many appropriate steps were taken to correct moisture intrusion and ventilation problems after the NIOSH visit. We understand that these were insufficient to prevent ongoing symptoms in occupants of the building, who have moved to another location.

RECOMMENDATIONS

Based on our findings, we recommend the actions listed below to create a more healthful workplace for future tenants.

Administrative Controls

Administrative controls are management-dictated work practices and policies to reduce or prevent exposures to workplace hazards. The effectiveness of administrative changes in work practices for controlling workplace hazards is dependent on management commitment and employee acceptance. Regular monitoring and reinforcement is necessary to ensure that control policies and procedures are not circumvented in the name of convenience or production efficiency.

1. Use track off floor mats at each door way.

2. Avoid the use of chair mats. If not feasible, use perforated floor mats.

3. As much as possible, keep papers and boxes off the floor. A non-cluttered room is easier to clean and HEPA vacuum. If feasible, an empty office could be converted into a storage area with shelves for boxes and filing cabinets for paper work.

4. Carpets should be routinely HEPA vacuumed. Ensure the HEPA-vacuum is well-maintained, and the HEPA filter is changed according to the manufacturer's recommendations. Avoid the use of carpet biocides.

5. We recommend carpet dust sampling to determine if carpet cleaning has been successful. The results can be compared

with the NIOSH carpet dust sample results collected in June 2011. If there is not a significant decrease in microbes, the carpet may need to be removed. If the carpet is replaced, we recommend monitoring the concrete slab for moisture intrusion rates in additional places beyond the previous moisture concrete slab testing.

6. Do not rely upon air sampling for mold since air concentrations cannot be interpreted with respect to health risk. Observing or smelling mold is sufficient motivation for dampness remediation when occupants have building-related symptoms.

7. Following the manufacturer's recommended maintenance schedules for the HVAC system, including replacing air filters, checking drip pans, ensuring thermostats are in working order, and checking and cleaning ventilation system dampers to ensure proper functioning.

8. Operate the ventilation system on a reduced setting (warmer during cooling months and cooler during heating months) during unoccupied hours instead of turning the system completely off.

9. Avoid using portable air cleaners that produce ozone, which can cause adverse respiratory effects. Information about ozone generators sold as air cleaners can be found on the U.S. EPA website at http://www.epa.gov/iaq/pubs/ozonegen.html.

10. Continue to routinely assess the building for water intrusion and damage and high relative humidity and correct these upon discovery. During and after heavy rains, walk through the building and check for water incursion. When sources of moisture are identified, repairs should be made to prevent further water entry into the building.

11. If there are continued health complaints by building occupants or musty or moldy odors, evaluate the area for hidden dampness and mold. An infrared camera can be used inside and outside the building after a heavy rain to look for hidden moisture and leaks. Also check for hidden sources under carpet (especially underneath windows or other areas with a history of leaking), above the ceiling, and in the walls (by cutting a hole in the wall and visually inspecting the area for odors, visible mold, and water damage).

RECOMMENDATIONS
(CONTINUED)

12. Any future mold and moisture-damaged materials should be promptly removed or cleaned with appropriate containment to minimize exposure for remediation workers, building occupants, and unaffected sections of the building. Keep a record of when and where mold or water-damaged materials are discovered and what has been done to promptly fix the underlying problem leading to the water damage.

13. Any building occupant who experiences worsening, persistent, or recurrent respiratory or other health symptoms that may be associated with being in the building should see his/her physician; the building occupant may need to be relocated to another site within the building or relocated to a different site out of the building.

14. Although there were no specific complaints about fragrance or colognes, consider implementing a fragrance-free policy.

References

American National Standards Institute (ANSI)/ASHRAE [2010A]. Thermal Environmental Conditions for Human Occupancy, standard 55-2010. American Society of Heating, Refrigeration, and Air-Conditioning Engineers, Atlanta, GA.

American National Standards Institute (ANSI)/ASHRAE [2010B]. Ventilation for acceptable indoor air quality, standard 62.1-2010. American Society of Heating, Refrigeration, and Air-Conditioning Engineers, Atlanta, GA.

Baldwin CM, Bell IR, O'Rourke MK [1999]. Odor sensitivity and respiratory complaint profiles in a community-based sample with asthma, hay fever, and chemical odor intolerance. Toxicol Ind Health 15:403–409.

Bridges B [2002]. Fragrance: emerging health and environmental concerns. Flavour Fragr J 17(5):361-371.

Buckley DA, Rycroft RJ, White IR, McFadden JP [2002]. Fragrance as an occupational allergen. Occup Med (Lond) 52(1):13-6.

Burge HA, Su HJ, Spengler JD [1994]. Moisture, organisms, and health effects. In: Trechsel HR, ed. Moisture control in buildings: (MNL 18). ASTM International, pp. 84-90.

Burge H [2010]. When should I use bacterial analysis of dust? http://www.emlab.com/s/sampling/2010-08-Dust-Bacteria.html. Date accessed: April 2013.

Caress SM, Steinemann AC [2009]. Prevalence of fragrance sensitivity in the American population. J Environ Health 71(7):46-50.

Cox-Ganser JM, Park J-H, Kreiss K [2010]. Office workers and teachers. In: Environmental and Occupational Lung Disease, Tarlo SM, Cullinan P, and Nemery B, eds. Environmental and Occupational Lung Disease. Chichester, UK: John Wiley & Sons, Ltd, ch 23.

Cummings KJ, Fink JN, Vasudev M, Piacitelli C, Kreiss K [2013]. Vocal cord dysfunction related to water-damaged buildings. J Allergy Clin Immunol: In Practice 1(1):46-50.

Custovic A, Green R, Taggart SC, Smith A, Pickering CA, Chapman MD, Woodcock A [1994]. Domestic allergens in public places II: Dog (Can f1) and cockroach (Bla g 2) allergens in dust and mite, cat, dog and cockroach allergens in the air in public buildings. Clin Exp Allergy 26(11):1246-52.

Custovic A, Fletcher A, Pickering CA, Francis HC, Green R, Smith A, Chapman M, Woodcock A [1998]. Domestic allergens in public places III: house dust mite, cat, dog and cockroach allergens in British hospitals. Clin Exp Allergy 28(1):53-59.

Eduard W [2009]. Fungal spores: a critical review of the toxicological and epidemiological evidence as a basis for occupational exposure limit setting. Crit Rev Toxicol 39(10):799-864.

Ebbehoj NE, Hansen MO, Sigsgaard T, Larsen L [2002]. Building-related symptoms and molds: a two-step intervention study. Indoor Air 12(4):273-277.

EPA (Environmental Protection Agency) [2008]. Mold remediation in schools and commercial buildings http://www.epa.gov/mold/mold_remediation.html. Date accessed: April 2013.

EPA [2009]. Residential air cleaners. Washington, DC: U.S. Department of Labor, Occupational Safety and Health Administration. EPA 402-F-09-002 (Revised August 2009) http://www.epa.gov/iaq/pubs/residair.html. Date assessed: April 2013.

EPA [2013]. Ozone generators that are sold as air cleaners http://www.epa.gov/iaq/pubs/ozonegen.html. Date assessed: April 2013.

Girard M, Israël-Assayag E, Cormier Y [2004]. Pathogenesis of hypersensitivity pneumonitis. Curr Opin Allergy Clin Immunol 4(2):93-98.

Haverinen-Shaughnessy U, Pekkanen J, Nevalainen A, Moschandreas D, Husman T [2004]. Estimating effects of moisture damage repairs on students' health-a long-term intervention study. J Expo Anal Environ Epidemiol 14 Suppl 1:S58-S64.

Haverinen-Shaughnessy U, Hyvärinen A, Putus T, Nevalainen A [2008] Monitoring success of remediation: seven case studies of moisture and mold damaged buildings. Sci Total Environ 399(1-3):19-27.

Hoy RF, Ribeiro M, Anderson J, Tarlo SM [2010]. Work-associated irritable larynx syndrome. Occup Med (Lond) 60(7):546-51.

Hung LL, Miller JD, Dillon HK, eds. [2005]. Field guide for the determination of biological contaminants in environmental samples. 2nd ed. Fairfax, VA: American Industrial Hygiene Association, pp. 29–38.

Institute of Medicine (IOM) [2004]. Institute of Medicine (IOM) [2004]. Damp indoor spaces and health. Washington, DC: National Academy of Sciences. Washington, DC: National Academy of Sciences.

Iossifova YY, Cox-Ganser JM, Park JH, White SK, Kreiss K [2011]. Lack of respiratory improvement following remediation of a water-damaged office building. Am J Ind Med 54(4):269-277.

Jarvis JQ, Morey PR [2001]. Allergic respiratory disease and fungal remediation in a building in a subtropical climate. Appl Occup Environ Hyg 16(3):380-388.

Kelman L [2004]. The premonitory symptoms (prodrome): a tertiary care study of 893 migraineurs. Headache 44(9):865-72.

Kelman L [2007]. The triggers or precipitants of the acute migraine attack. Cephalalgia 27(5):394–402.

Kercsmar CM, Dearborn DG, Schluchter M, Xue L, Kirchner HL, Sobolewski J, Greenberg SJ, Vesper SJ, Allan T [2006]. Reduction in asthma morbidity in children as a result of home remediation aimed at moisture sources. Environ Health Perspect 114(10):1574-1580.

Kumar P, Caradonna-Graham VM, Gupta S, Cai X, Rao PN, Thompson J [1995]. Inhalation challenge effects of perfume scent strips in patients with asthma. Ann Allergy Asthma Immunol 75(5):429-33.

Lignell U, Meklin T, Putus T, Rintala H, Vepsäläinen A, Kalliokoski P, Nevalainen A [2007]. Effects of moisture damage and renovation on microbial conditions and pupils' health in two schools: a longitudinal analysis of five years. J Environ Monit 9(3):225-233.

Meklin T, Potus T, Pekkanen J, Hyvärinen A, Hirvonen MR, Nevalainen A [2005]. Effects of moisture-damage repairs on microbial exposure and symptoms in school children. Indoor Air 15 Suppl 10:40.

Mendell MJ, Mirer AG, Cheung K, Tong M, Douwes J [2011]. Respiratory and allergic health effects of dampness, mold, and dampness-related agents: a review of the epidemiologic evidence. Environ Health Perspect 119(6):748-56.

OSHA [1999]. OSHA Technical Manual. Washington, DC: U.S. Department of Labor, Occupational Safety and Health Administration. Directive Number: TED 01-00-015 http://www.osha.gov/dts/osta/otm/otm_toc.html. Date accessed: April 2013.

Patovirta RL, Husman T, Haverinen U, Vahteristo M, Uitti JA, Tukiainen H, Nevalainen A [2004]. The remediation of mold damaged school–a three-year follow-up study on teachers' health. Cent Eur J Public Health 12(1):36-42.

Perfetti L, Ferrari M, Galdi E, Pozzi V, Cottica D, Grignani E, Minoia C, Moscato G [2004]. House dust mites (Der p 1, Der f 1), cat (Fel d 1) and cockroach (Bla g 2) allergens in indoor work-places (offices and archives). Sci Total Environ 26;328(1-3):15-21.

Prezant B, Weekes DM, Miller JD, eds. [2008]. Recognition, evaluation, and control of indoor mold. Virginia: American Industrial Hygiene Association.

Sesline D, Ames RG, Howd RA [1994]. Irritative and systemic symptoms following exposure to Microban disinfectant through a school ventilation system. Arch Environ Health 49(6):439–444.

World Health Organization (WHO) [2009]. WHO guidelines for indoor air quality: dampness and mould. WHO Regional Office for Europe.

Table 1. Air measurements obtained by NIOSH investigators on June 22, 2011, accounting office, Florida

Location		Time	Carbon Dioxide (ppm*)	Carbon Monoxide (ppm)	Hydrogen Sulfide (ppm)	Total VOCs* (ppm)		Temperature (°F)	Relative Humidity (%)
						PID*	FID*		
Outside	Front parking lot	14:34	416	0†	0†	0.2	2.0	88	65
Outside	Roof (multiple sites)	8:15‡	--	--	0	--	--	--	--
Room 1	Conference room	14:42	650	0.3	0	0.2	1.8	74	50
Room 2	Office	14:46	--	--	--	0.2	1.6	--	--
Cubicles	Near Room 2	14:45	655	0.2	0	0.2	1.6	74	54
Room 3	Office	14:47	618	0.2	0	0.1	1.5	72	55
Room 4	Office	14:52	680	0	0	0.1	1.5	72	57
Room 6	Office	14:54	684	0	0	0.1	1.4	72	55
Room 7	Office	14:57	--	--	--	0.1	1.4	--	--
Room 9	Office	15:20	626	0	0	0.1	1.5	72	55
Room 12	Office	15:18	647	0	0	0.1	1.4	73	58
Room 15	Office	15:15	632	0	0	0.1	1.4	73	56
Room 16	Office	15:14	651	0	0	0.1	1.4	72	59
Room 18	Office	15:12	651	0	0	0.1	1.4	72	57
Room 20	Office	15:10	634	0	0	0.1	1.4	71	57
Room 25	Office	15:08	640	0	0	0.1	1.4	72	55
Room 28	Reception	15:06	646	0	0	--	--	72	57
Room 29	Office	15:05	620	0	0	0.1	1.4	72	56
Room 30	Office	15:02	605	0	0	0.1	1.4	73	58
Room 31	Office	15:04	621	0	0	--	--	73	61
Room 34	Reception	14:59	637	0	0	0.2	1.6	73	58
Room 36	Office	14:57	652	0	0	0.1	1.4	72	59
Room 38	Storage	15:24	--	--	--	0.1	1.5	--	--
Average inside			642	0.04	0	0.1	1.5	72	56
Minimum inside			605	0	0	0.1	1.4	71	50
Maximum inside			684	0.3	0	0.2	1.8	74	61

* ppm = parts contaminant per million parts air; VOC = volatile organic compound; PID = photoionization detector; FID = flame ionization detector; -- (dashes) = not sampled

† detection limit 0.1 ppm; ‡ samples collected on June 23, 2011

Table 2. Microbial agents cultured* from carpet dust vacuum samples collected by NIOSH investigators on June 22, 2011, accounting office, Florida

Sample location	Fungi		Bacteria	
	Identification	cfu/g†	Identification	cfu/g†
Room 2	*Alternaria alternata*	1,200	*Bacillus*	440,000
	Aspergillus niger	1,600	Gram negative rods	1,300,000
	Aureobasidium pullulans	800	Gram positive cocci	40,000
	Basidiomycetes	800	Total bacteria	1,800,000
	Cladosporium cladosporioides	1,200		
	Curvularia lunata	400	Thermophilic actinomycetes	800
	Epicoccum nigrum	2,000		
	Nonsporulating Fungi	800		
	Penicillium minioluteum	400		
	Penicillium sclerotiorum	400		
	Pithomyces chartarum	1,200		
	Yeasts	1,200		
	Total fungi	12,000		
Hall 5 (by SW back door)	*Aspergillus ochraceus*	80,000	*Bacillus*	800,000
	Aspergillus sydowii	80,000	Gram negative rods	99,000,000
	Aspergillus ustus	1,800,000	Total bacteria	100,000,000
	Basidiomycetes	80,000		
	Cladosporium cladosporioides	160,000	Thermophilic actinomycetes	2,800
	Penicillium chrysogenum	320,000		
	Total fungi	2,500,000		
Hall 5 (between Room 4 and hallway)	*Alternaria alternata*	4,000	*Bacillus*	120,000
	Aspergillus niger	4,000	Gram negative rods	4,600,000
	Aspergillus ustus	56,000	Total bacteria	4,800,000
	Fusarium species	12,000		
	Yeast	20,000	Thermophilic actinomycetes	1,600
	Total fungi	96,000		
Room 6	*Alternaria alternata*	4,000	*Bacillus*	68,000
	Aspergillus niger	24,000	Gram negative rods	160,000
	Aspergillus ustus	8,000	Total bacteria	220,000
	Basidiomycete	8,000		
	Chaetomium globosum	8,000	Thermophilic actinomycetes	1,600
	Cladosporium cladosporioides	8,000		
	Curvularia lunata	8,000		
	Nonsporulating fungi	16,000		
	Total fungi	84,000		

Tables (continued)

Table 2 (continued). Microbial agents cultured* from carpet dust vacuum samples collected by NIOSH investigators on June 22, 2011, accounting office, Florida

Sample location	Fungi		Bacteria	
	Identification	cfu/g†	Identification	cfu/g†
Hall 11 (by middle back door)	Aspergillus ustus	20,000	Bacillus	800,000
	Cladosporium cladosporioides	24,000	Gram negative rods	23,000,000
	Nonsporulating fungi	20,000	Gram positive cocci	400,000
	Paecilomyces marquandii	4,000	Total bacteria	24,000,000
	Penicillium brevicompactum	4,000		
	Penicillium chrysogenum	4,000	Thermophilic actinomycetes	400
	Phoma species	350,000		
	Total fungi	420,000		
Room 12	Aspergillus caespitosus	4,000	Bacillus	40,000
	Aspergillus flavus	8,000	Gram negative rods	2,800,000
	Aspergillus niger	24,000	Gram negative cocci	1,200,000
	Aspergillus ochraceus	8,000	Total bacteria	4,000,000
	Cladosporium cladosporioides	4,000		
	Curvularia lunata	4,000	Thermophilic actinomycetes	<400
	Nonsporulating fungi	28,000		
	Yeast	8,000		
	Total fungi	88,000		
Storage area (by Room 25)	Alternaria alternata	4,000	Bacillus	38,000
	Aspergillus caespitosus	8,000	Gram negative rods	2,800
	Aspergillus niger	12,000	Total bacteria	41,000
	Aspergillus sydowii	12,000		
	Aspergillus ustus	28,000	Thermophilic actinomycetes	1,200
	Penicillium brevicompactum	320,000		
	Penicillium species	4,000		
	Total fungi	390,000		
Room 29	Aspergillus niger	32,000	Actinomycetes	16,000
	Curvularia lunata	4,000	Bacillus	84,000
	Nonsporulating fungi	8,000	Gram negative rods	48,000
	Phoma species	36,000	Gram positive cocci	36,000
	Yeast	4,000	Total bacteria	180,000
	Total fungi	84,000		
			Thermophilic actinomycetes	1,200
Room 31	Aspergillus ochraceus	180,000	Actinomycetes	400
	Nonsporulating fungi	4,000	Bacillus	18,000
	Yeast	4,000	Gram negative rods	6,000
	Total fungi	190,000	Gram positive cocci	400
			Total bacteria	25,000
			Thermophilic actinomycetes	400

* Fungi cultured on malt extract agar (MEA) media at 23-26°C; bacteria cultured on tryptic soy agar (TSA) media at 23-26°C, except thermophilic actinomycetes bacteria cultured at 55°C.
†cfu/g = colony forming units per gram.

Table 3. Microbial agents cultured* from bulk material samples collected from inside ventilation insulation board supply ducts by NIOSH investigators on June 22, 2011, accounting office, Florida

Sample Description	Fungi		Bacteria	
	Identification	cfu/g†	Identification	cfu/g†
BLK 10 Cutout sample from HVAC-1 supply duct above Room 3	*Cladosporium cladosporioides*	120,000	*Bacillus*	1,000
	Verticillium lecanii	38,000	*Gram negative rods*	400
	Total fungi	158,000	Total bacteria	1,400
			Thermophilic actinomycetes	<100
BLK 11 Cutout sample from HVAC-4 supply duct above hallway by Room 12	*Acrodontium* species	9,200,000	*Bacillus*	700
	Cladosporium cladosporioides	100,000	Total bacteria	700
	Total fungi	9,300,000		
			Thermophilic actinomycetes	<100

*Fungi cultured on malt extract agar (MEA) media at 23-26°C; bacteria cultured on tryptic soy agar (TSA) media at 23-26°C, except thermophilic actinomycetes bacteria cultured at 55°C.
†cfu/g = colony forming units per gram.

Table 4. Microbial agents identified with direct microscopic examination in bulk material samples collected from inside ventilation insulation board supply ducts by NIOSH investigators on June 22, 2011, accounting office, Florida

Sample Description	Mold growth seen with underlying mycelial and/or sporulating structures*		Miscellaneous spores present†	General Impression
BLK 10 Cutout sample from HVAC-1 supply duct above Room 3	2+	*Sporothrix* species (spores, hyphae, conidiophores)	None	Mold growth
	2+	*Cladosporium* species (spores, hyphae, conidiophores)		
BLK 12 Tape lift sample from AHU-1 supply duct on roof	4+	*Sporothrix* species (spores, hyphae, conidiophores)	None	Mold growth
	4+	*Cladosporium* species (spores, hyphae, conidiophores)		
BLK 11 Cutout sample from HVAC-4 supply duct above hallway by Room 12	3+	*Sporothrix* species (spores, hyphae, conidiophores)	None	Mold growth
	1+	*Cladosporium* species (spores, hyphae, conidiophores)		
BLK 14 Tape lift sample from HVAC-4 supply duct above hallway by Room 12	4+	*Sporothrix* species (spores, hyphae, conidiophores)	None	Mold growth
	1+	*Cladosporium* species (spores, hyphae, conidiophores)		
BLK 16 Tweezed sample from HVAC-4 supply duct above hallway by Room 12	4+	*Sporothrix* species (spores, hyphae, conidiophores)	None	Mold growth
	3+	*Cladosporium* species (spores, hyphae, conidiophores)		
BLK 13 Tape lift sample from AHU-4 supply duct on roof	4+	*Sporothrix* species (spores, hyphae, conidiophores)	None	Mold growth
	1+	*Cladosporium* species (spores, hyphae, conidiophores)		
BLK 15 Tweezed sample from AHU-4 supply duct on roof	4+	*Sporothrix* species (spores, hyphae, conidiophores)	None	Mold growth
	3+	*Cladosporium* species (spores, hyphae, conidiophores)		

* Quantities of molds are graded 1+ to 4+, with 4+ denoting the highest numbers.
†Indicative of normal conditions (i.e., seen on surfaces everywhere), including basidiospores (mushroom spores), myxomycetes, plant pathogens such as ascospores, rusts and smuts, and a mix of saprophytic genera with no particular spore type predominating and a distribution of spore types usually seen outdoors

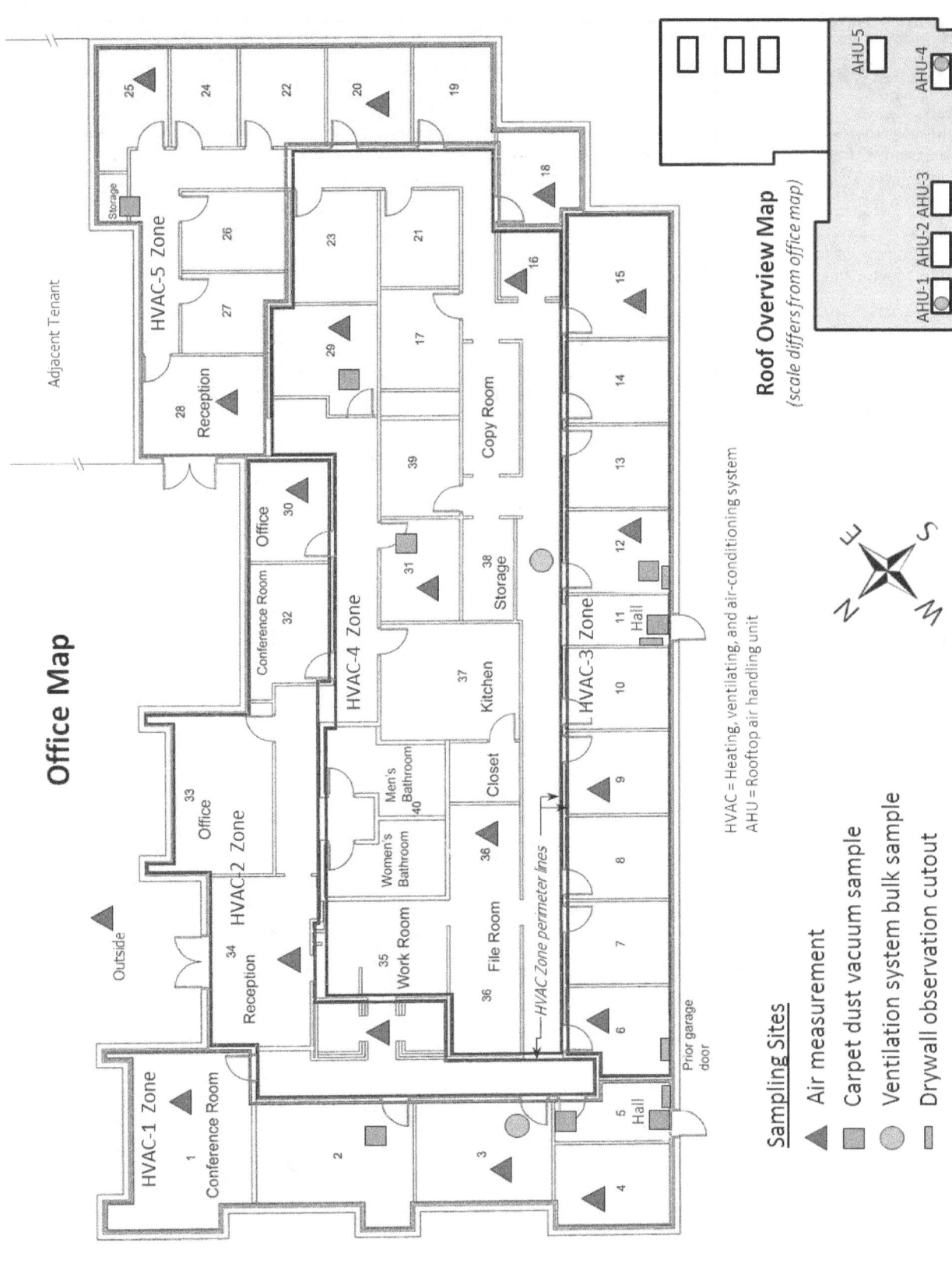

Figure 1. Map with sampling locations.

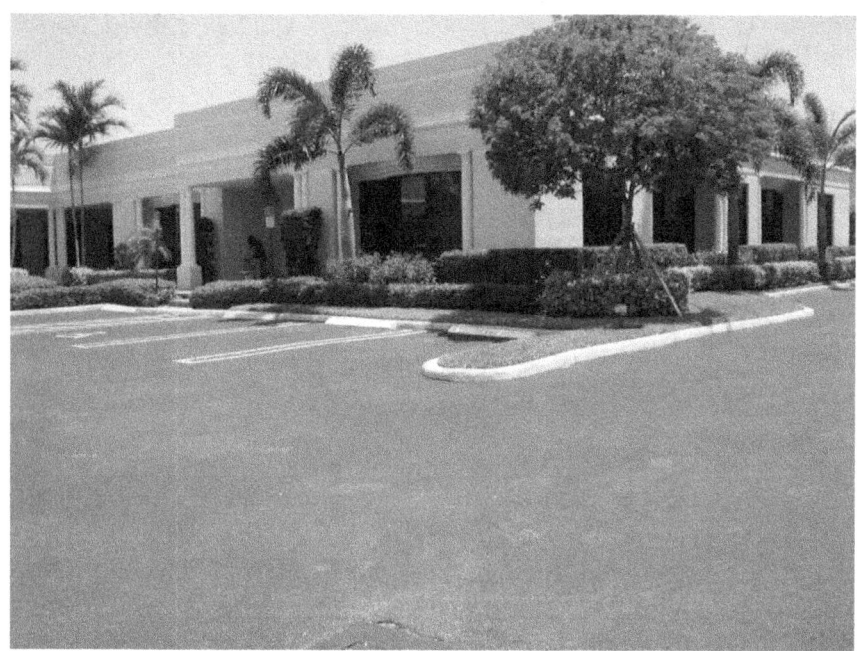

Figure 2. Exterior of front of office building, June 2011.

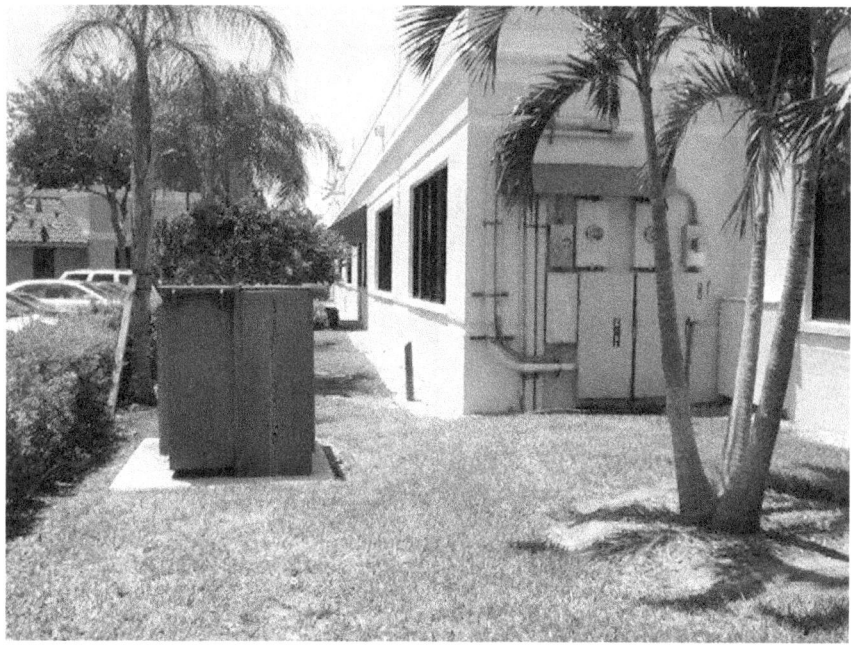

Figure 3. Exterior of back of office building, June 2011.

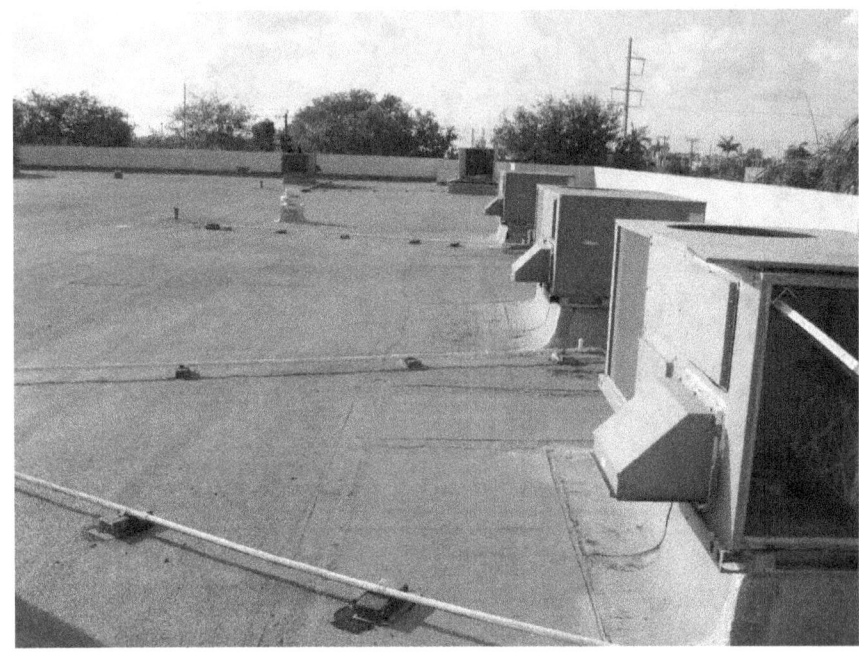

Figure 4. Roof-top air-handling units 1 (foreground) through 5 with condensate pipes that extend to roof drains, June 2011.

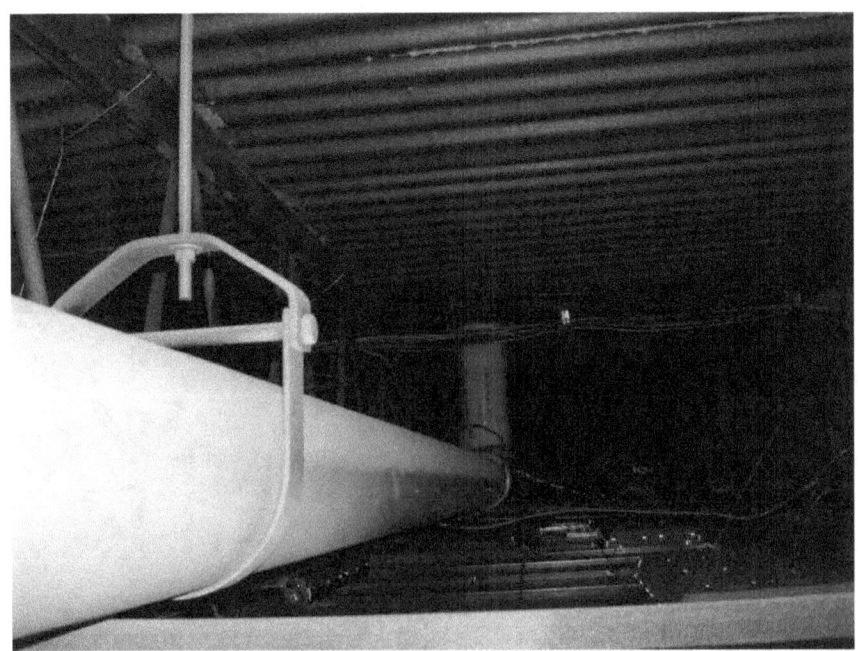

Figure 5. Roof drainpipe inside ceiling plenum, June 2011.

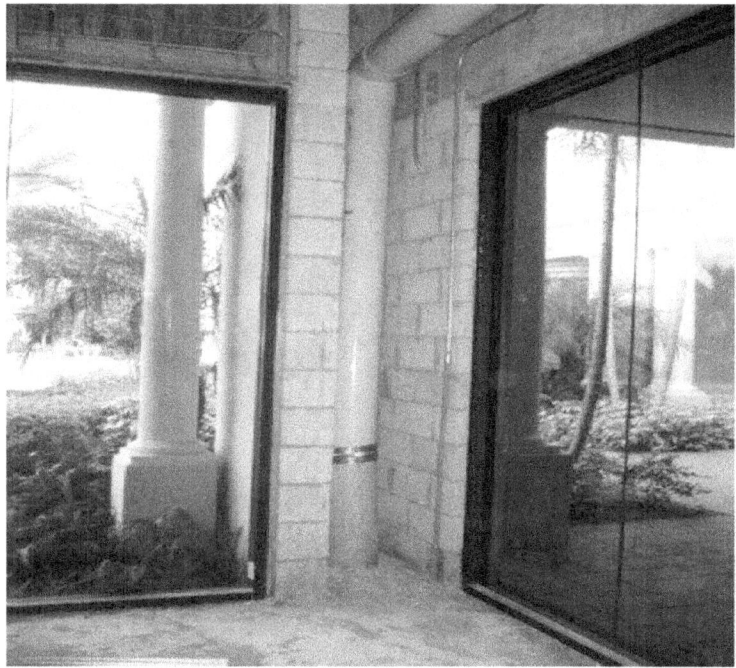

Figure 6. Roof drainpipe dropped through the exterior wall (exposed during 2006-7 renovation) into the ground, October 2006 (picture courtesy of building manager).

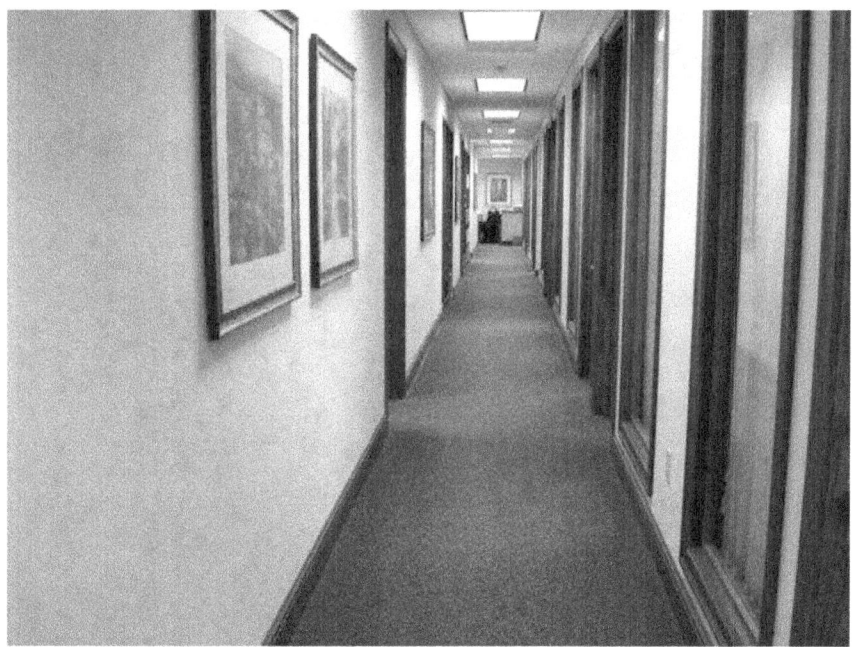

Figure 7. Hallway inside accounting office, June 2011.

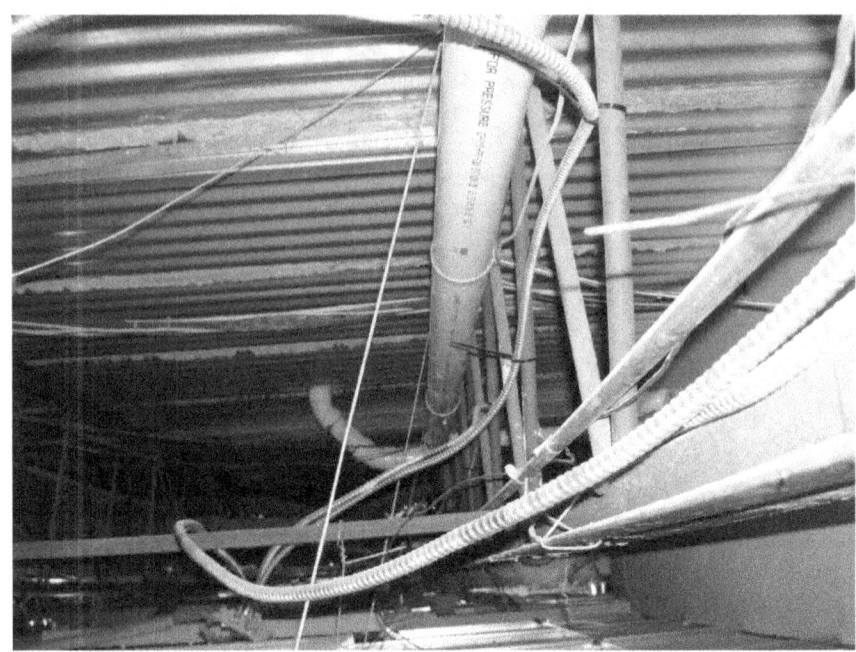

Figure 8. Ceiling plenum, June 2011.

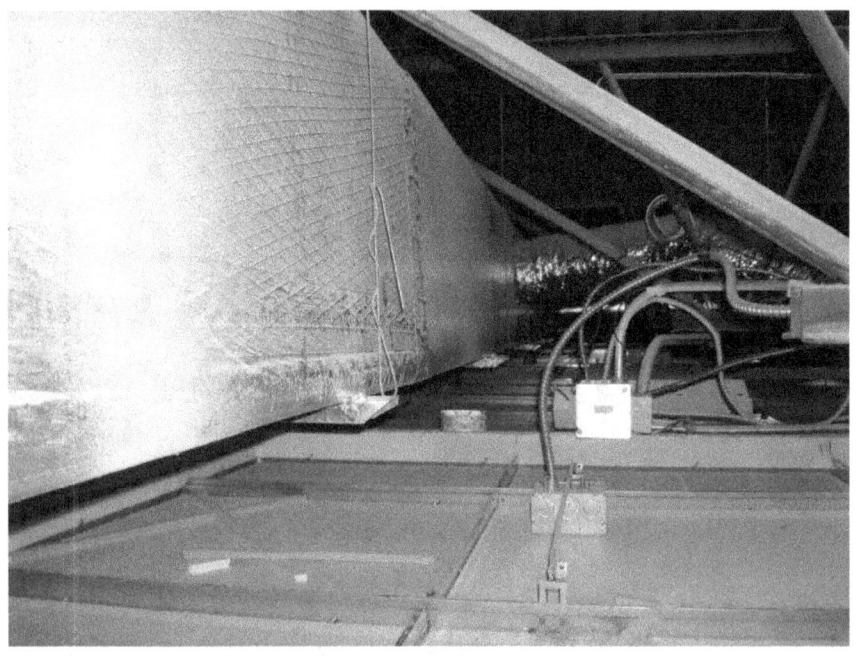

Figure 9. HVAC main trunk line, June 2011.

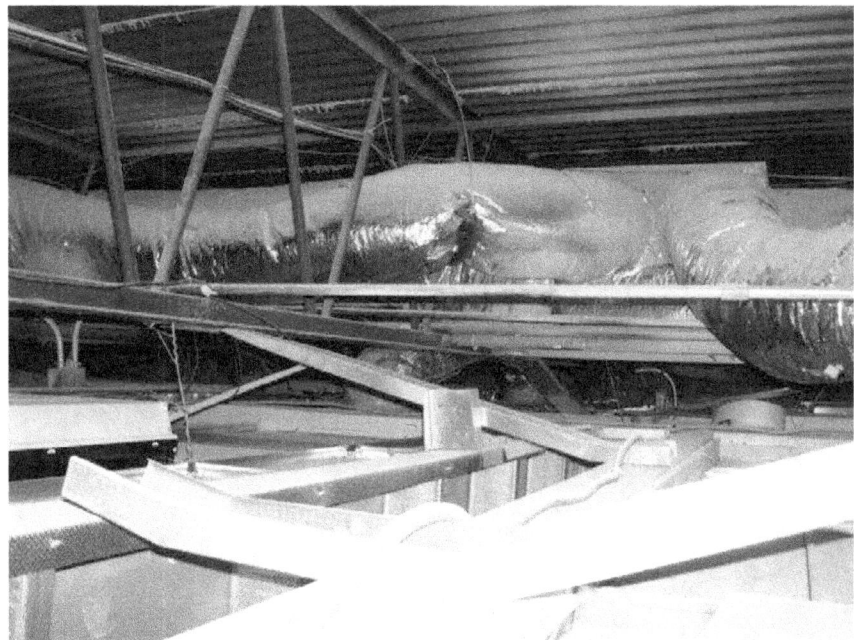

Figure 10. HVAC main trunk line with multiple flexible ducts attached, June 2011.

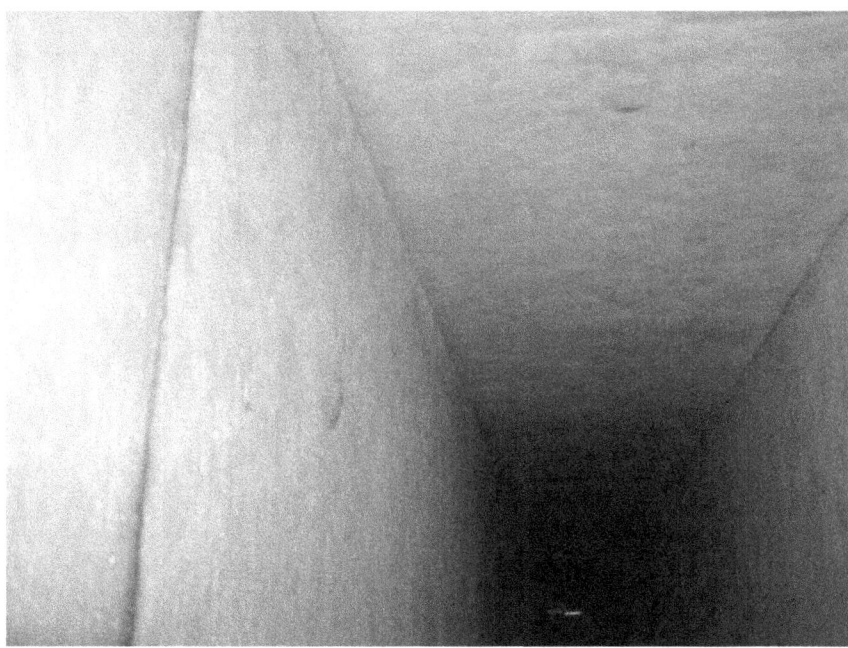

Figure 11. Inside of an HVAC main trunk line, June 2011.

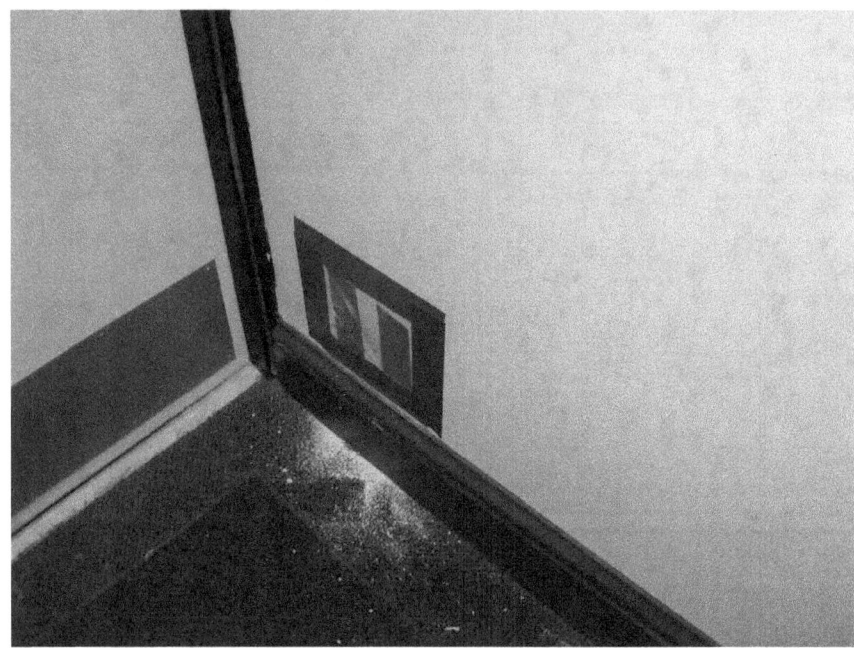

Figure 12. Wall cavity inspection hole after sealing with tape in Hall 11 wall shared with Room 10, June 2011.

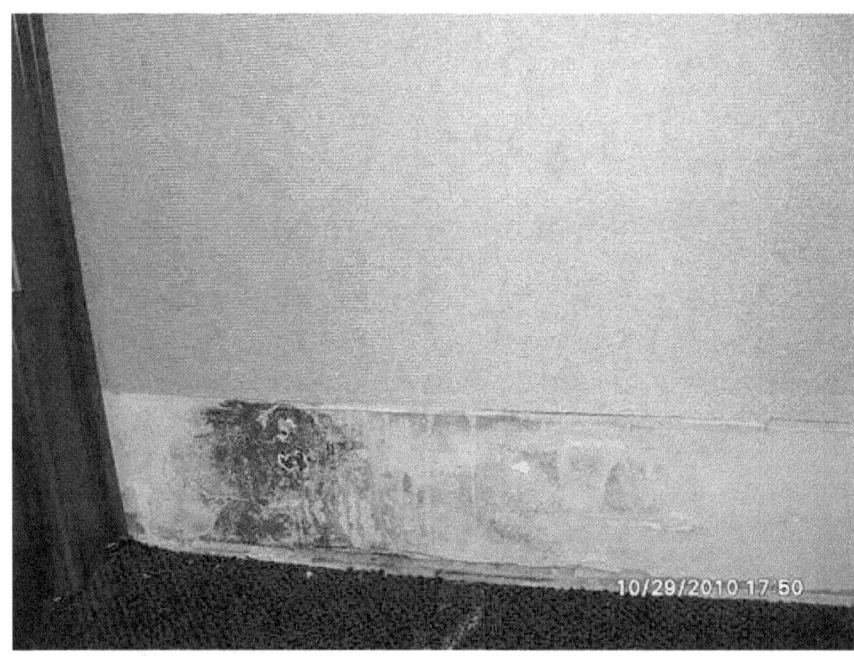

Figure 13. Suspect mold in Room 3 at base of wall shared with Hall 5, October 2010 (picture courtesy of building manager).

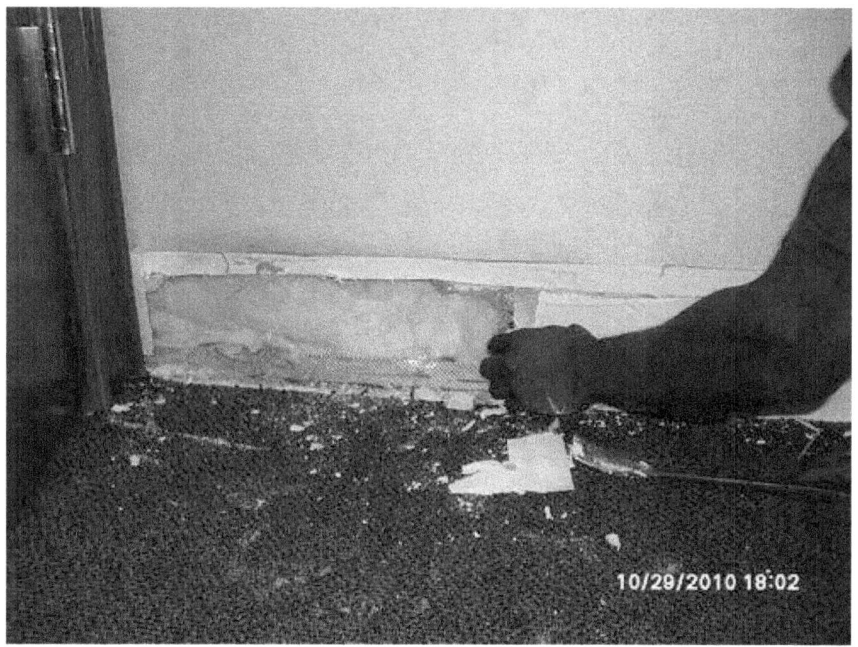

Figure 14. Suspect mold-damaged drywall removed in Room 3 at base of wall shared with Hall 5, October 2010 (picture courtesy of building manager).

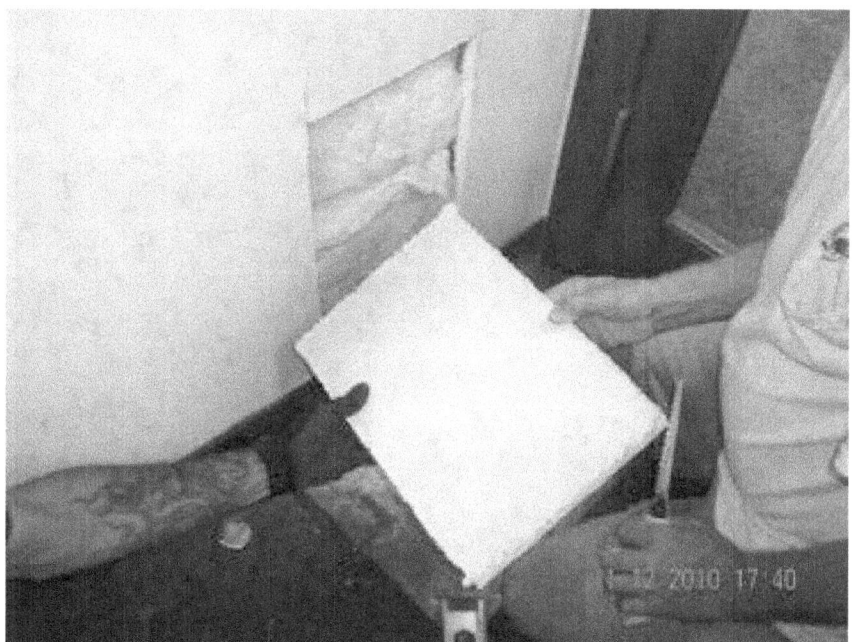

Figure 15. Wall cavity inspection inside Hall 5 wall shared with Room 3, November 2010 (picture courtesy of building manager).

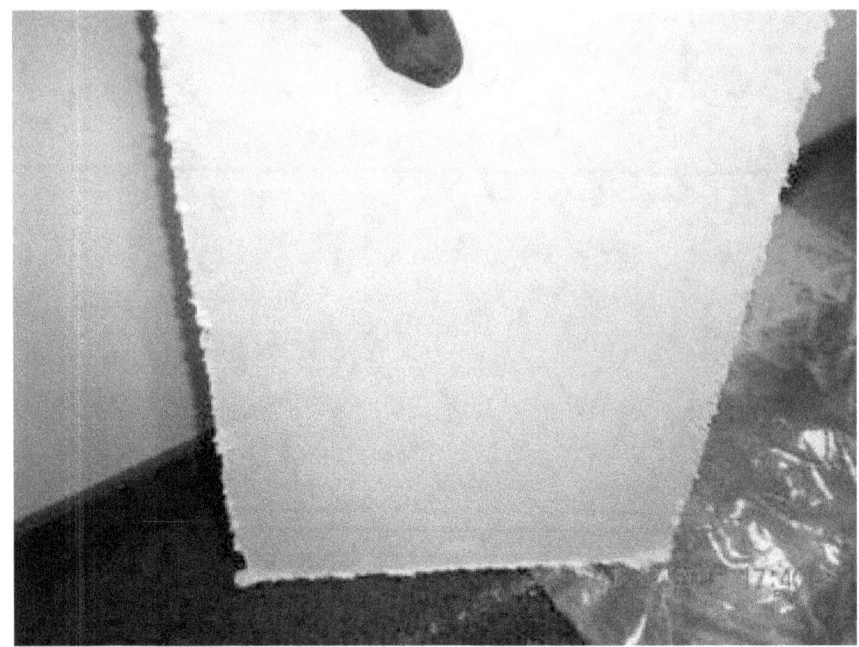

Figure 16. Wall cavity inspection, November 2010 (picture courtesy of building manager).

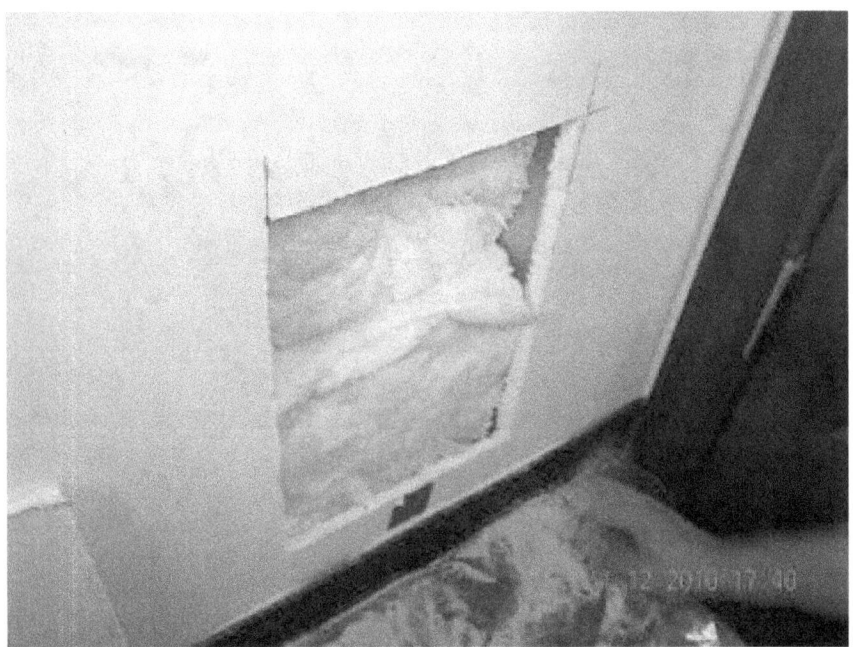

Figure 17. Wall cavity inspection inside Hall 5 wall shared with Room 3, November 2010 (picture courtesy of building manager).

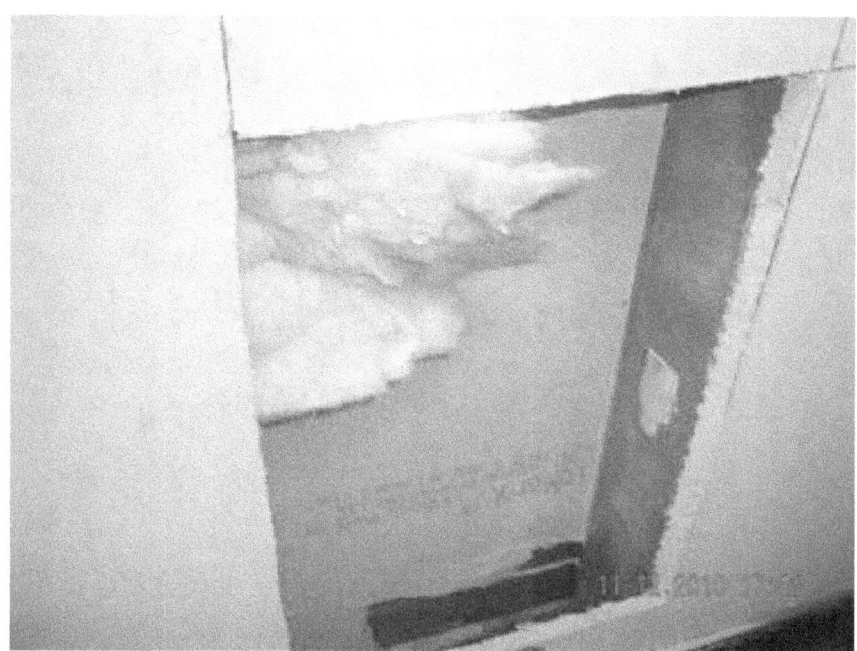

Figure 18. Wall cavity inspection inside Hall 5 wall shared with Room 3, November 2010 (picture courtesy of building manager).

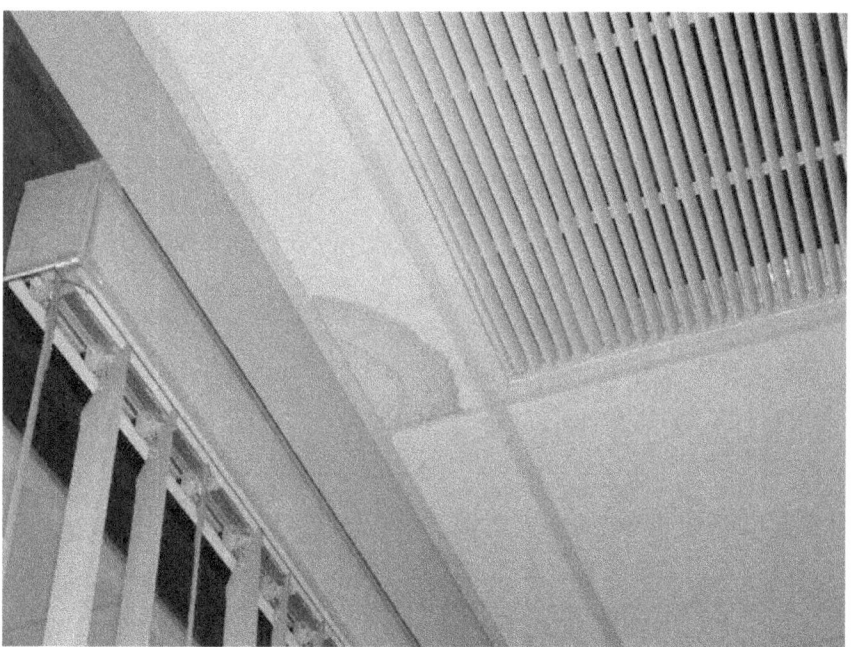

Figure 19. Ceiling stain in Room 23, June 2011.

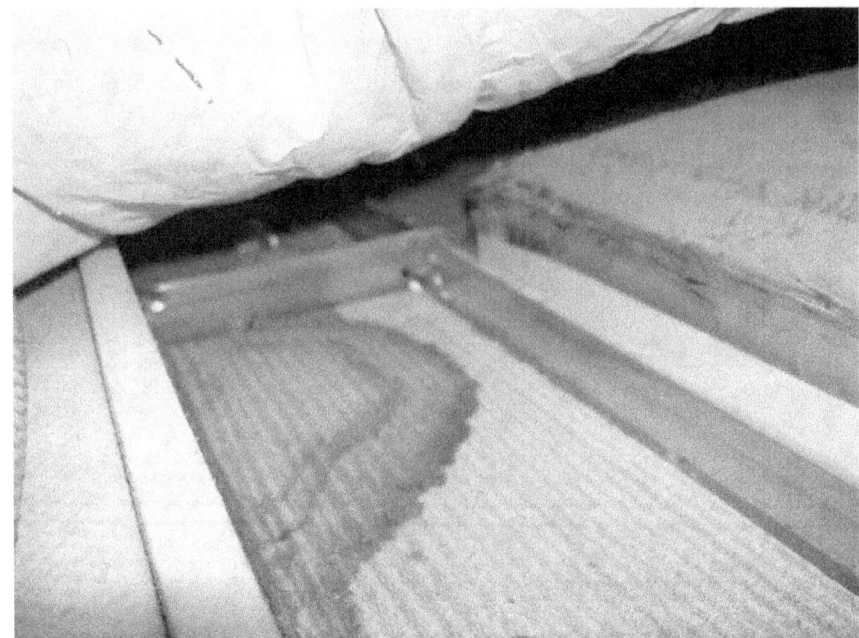

Figure 20. Top of stained ceiling tile in Room 23, June 2011.

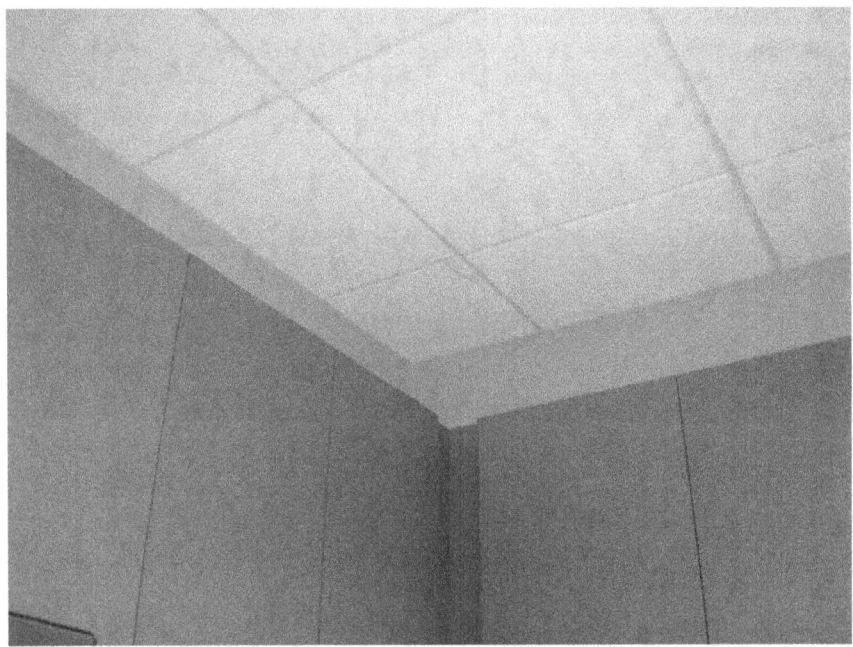

Figure 21. Ceiling stain in Room 37 (kitchen), June 2011.

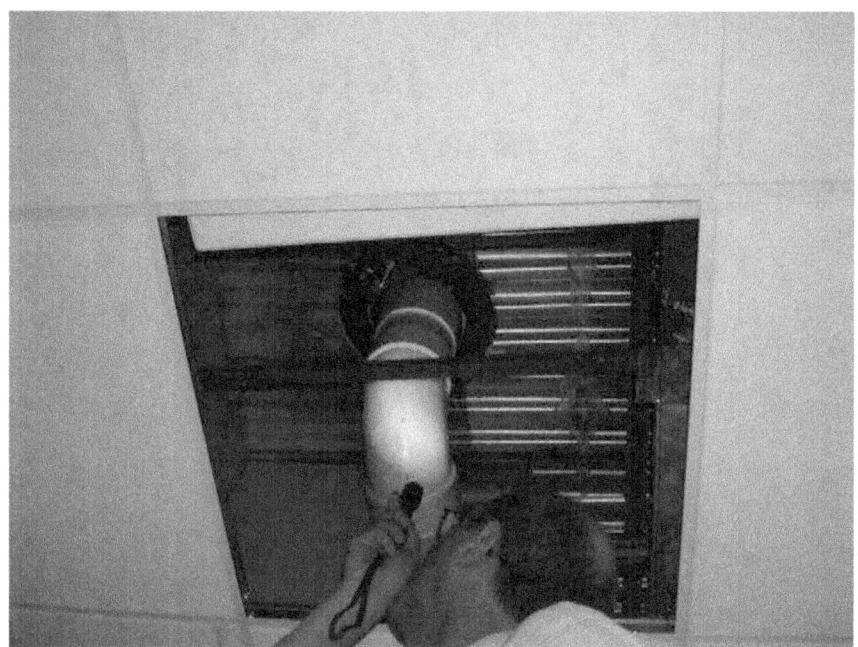

Figure 22. Roof drain above ceiling stain in Room 37 (kitchen), June 2011.

Figure 23. Raised area of cloth wall paper in Room 3, June 2011.

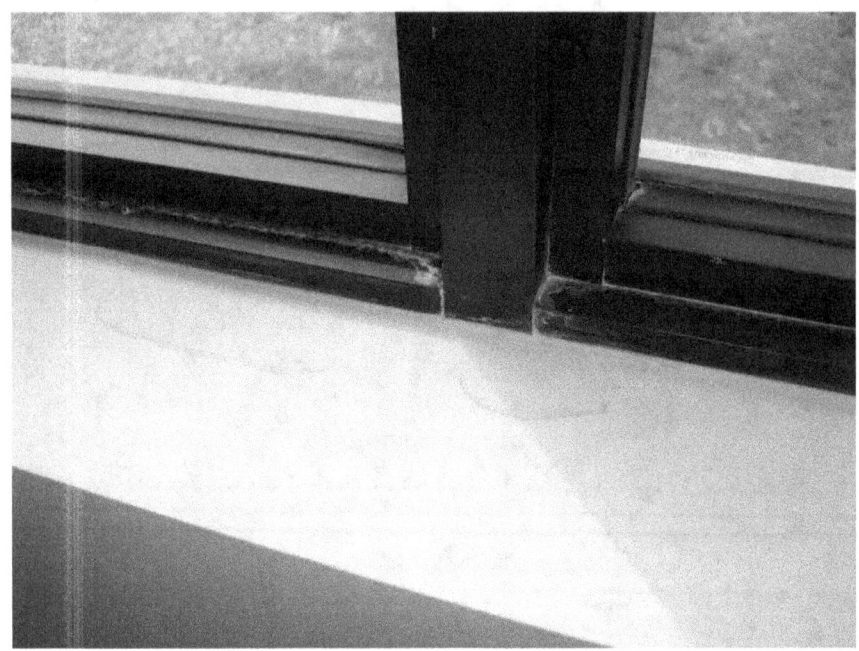

Figure 24. Water stains on window sill in Room 19, June 2011.

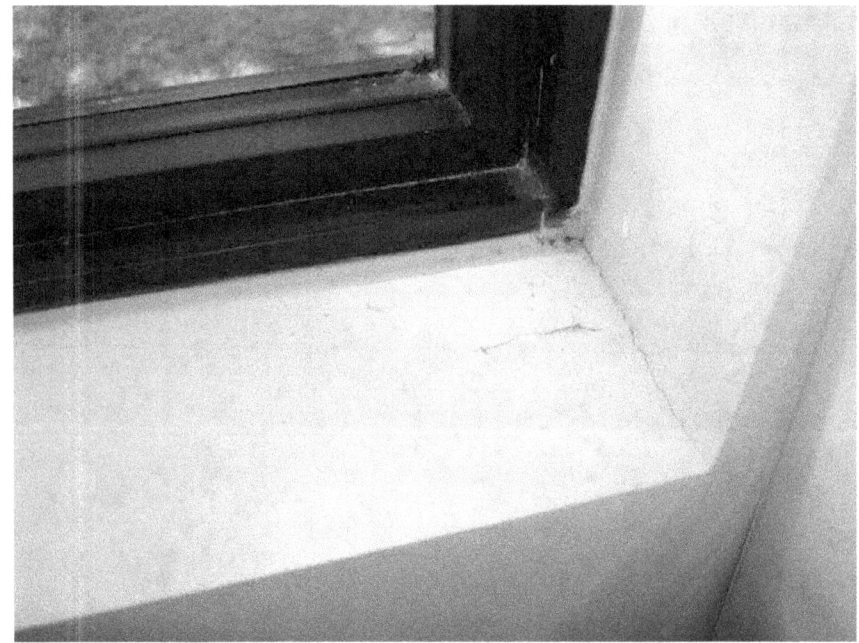

Figure 25. Blistered paint on window sill in Room 19, June 2011.

Figure 26. Vertical water marks on wall under window in Hall 11, June 2011.

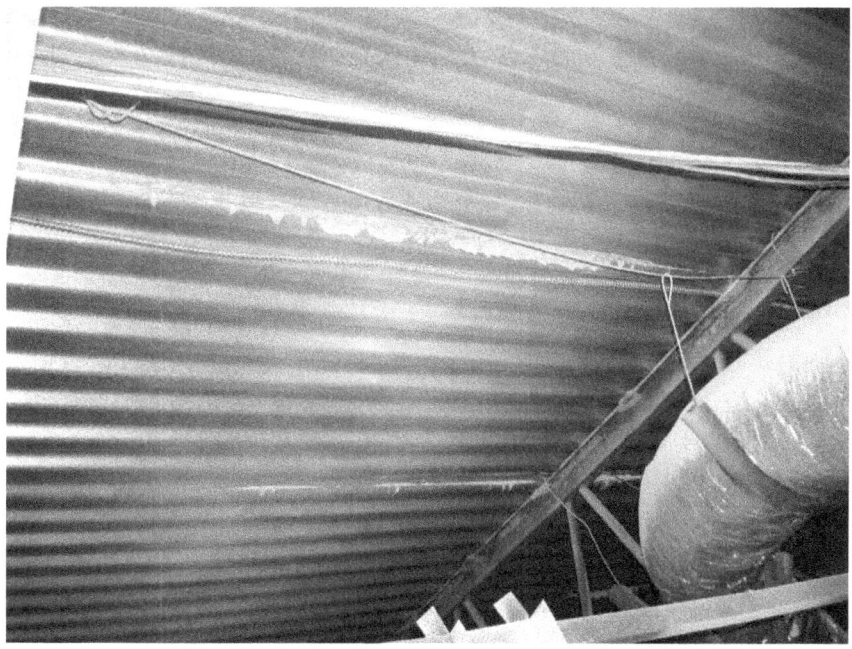

Figure 27. Roof lap joints inside ceiling plenum, June 2011.

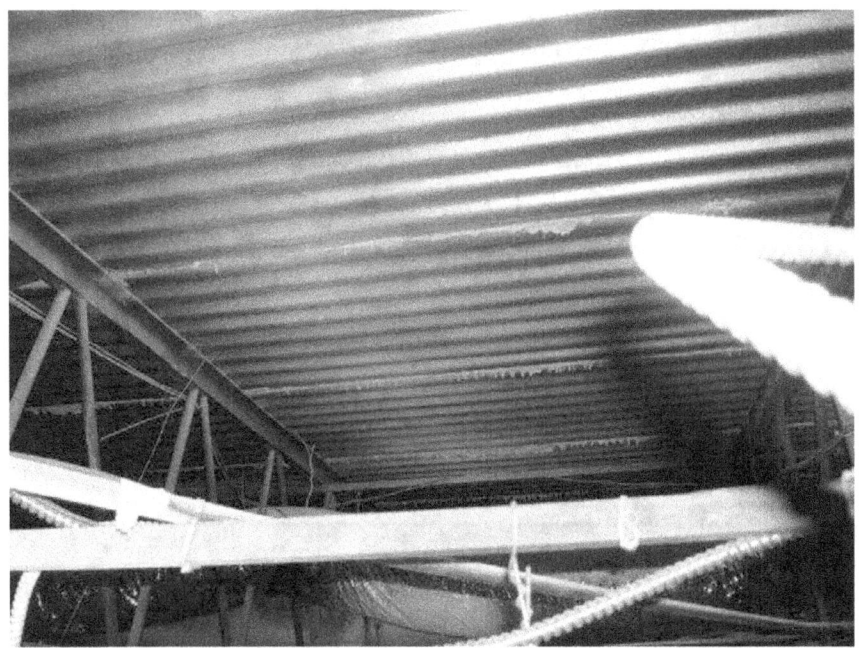

Figure 28. Roof lap joints inside ceiling plenum, June 2011.

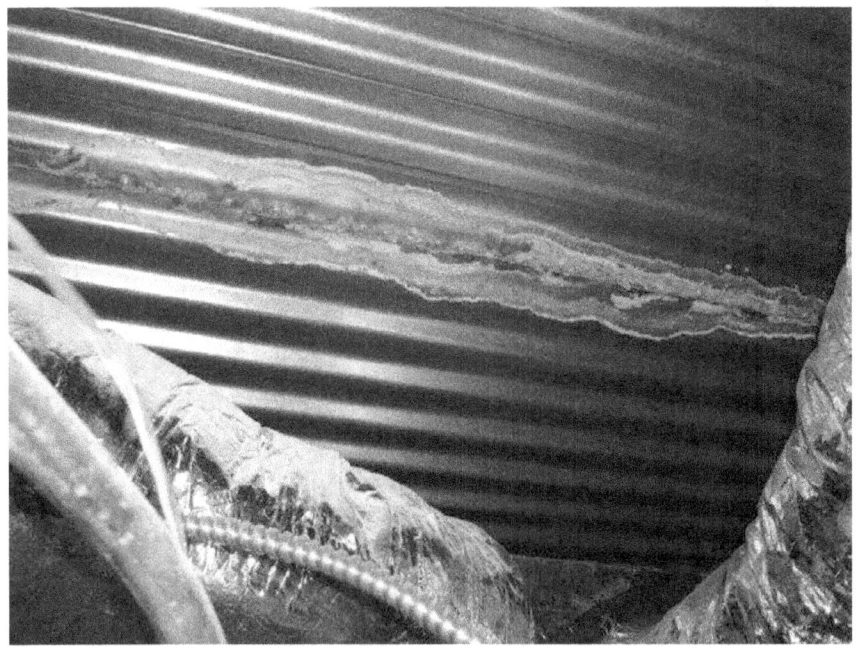

Figure 29. Rusty stain at a roof lap joint in ceiling plenum, June 2011.

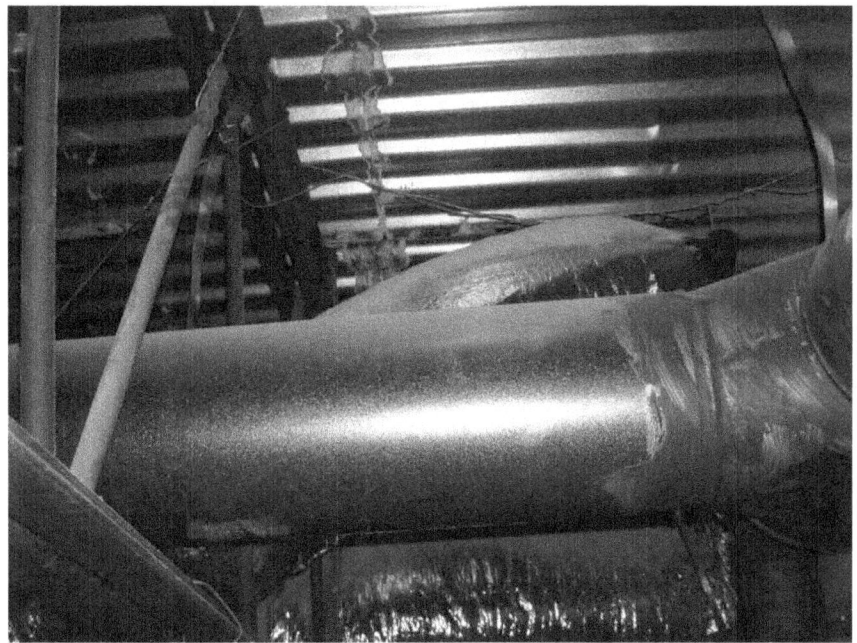

Figure 30. Rusty stain at a roof lap joint in ceiling plenum, June 2011.

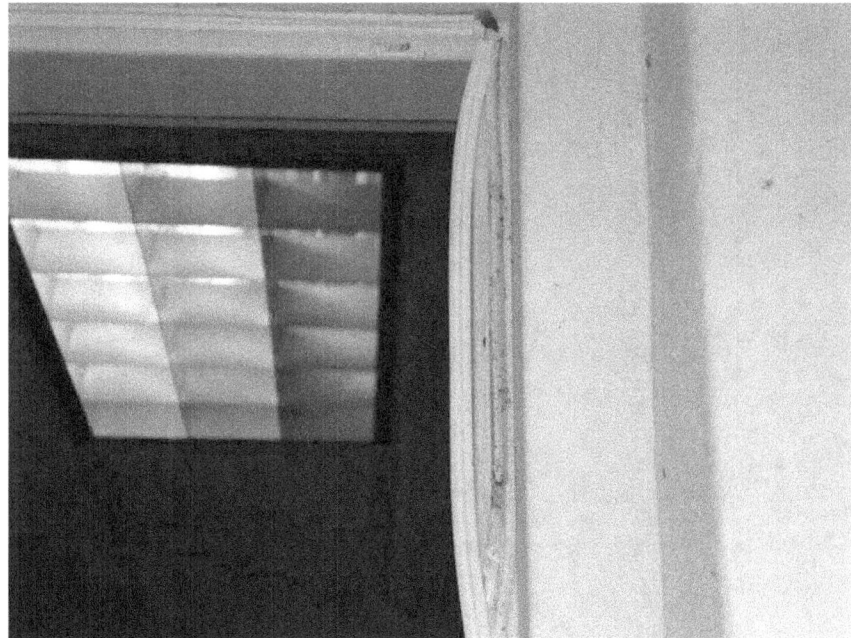

Figure 31. Ill-fitting weather stripping on Hall 5 exterior door frame, June 2011.

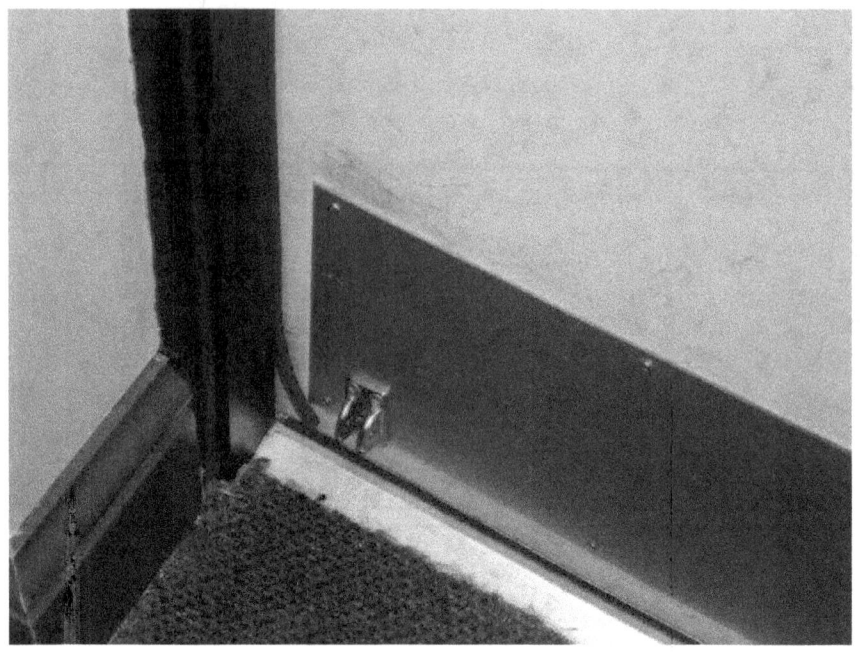

Figure 32. Ill-fitting weather stripping on door frame in Hall 5, June 2011.

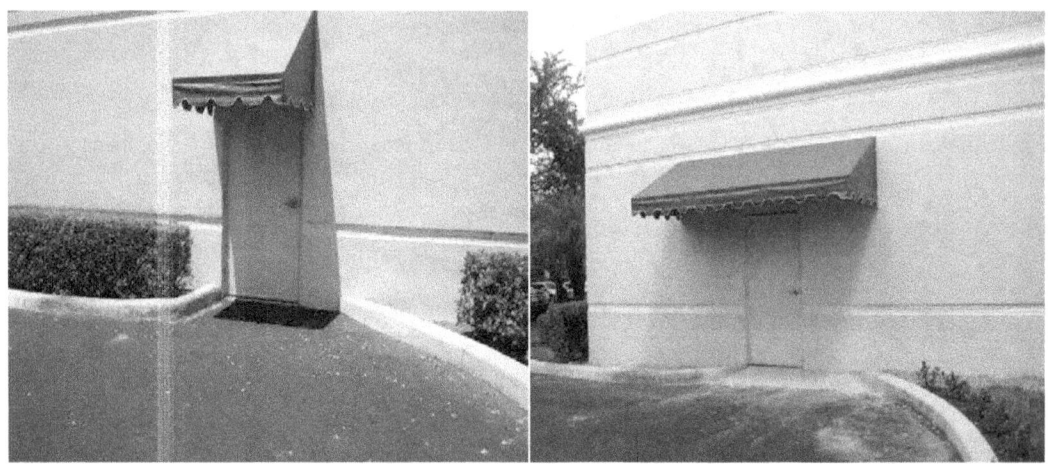

Figure 33. Awning over Hall 5 exterior door
a) June 2011.   b) September 2011 (courtesy of building manager).

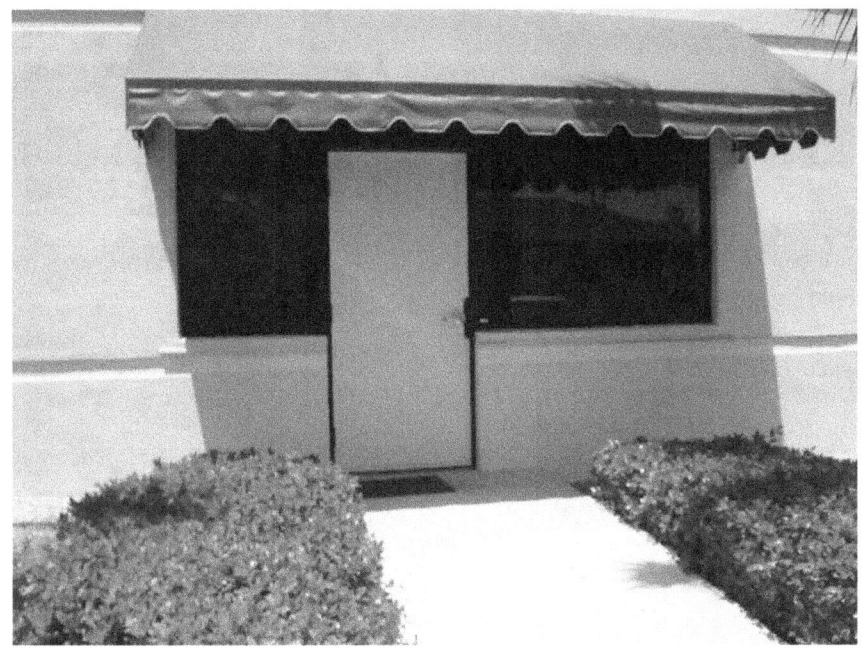

Figure 34. Awning over Hall 11 exterior door, June 2011.

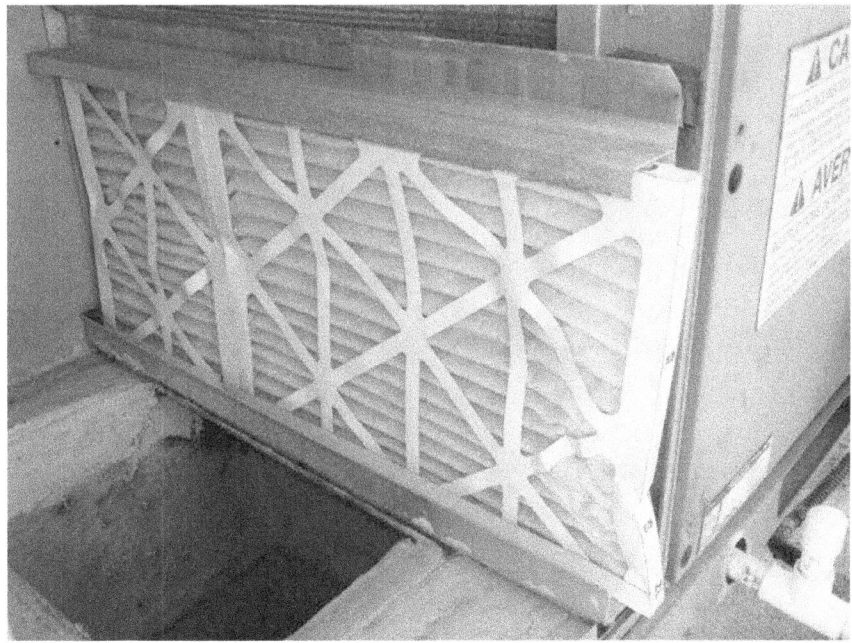

Figure 35. Oversized filter in AHU-2, June 2011.

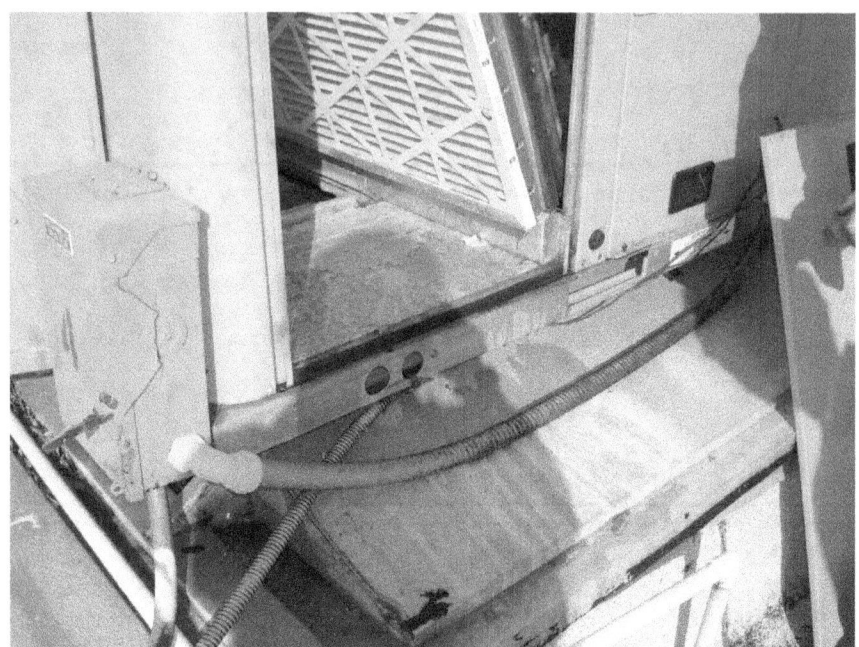

Figure 36. Water dripping into AHU-4 filter housing base and outside/return air mixing plenum, June 2011.

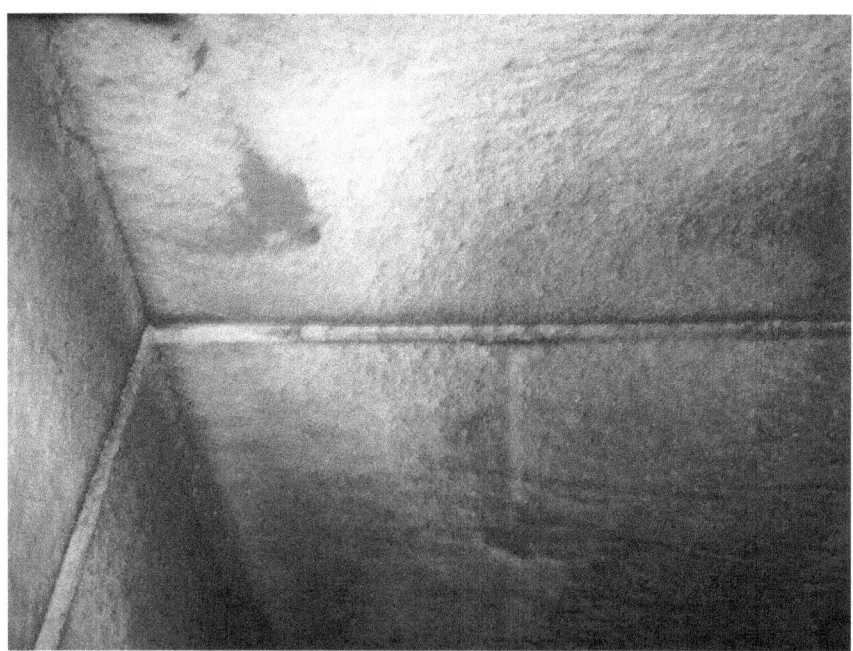

Figure 37. Inside supply duct immediately after fan in AHU-1, June 2011.

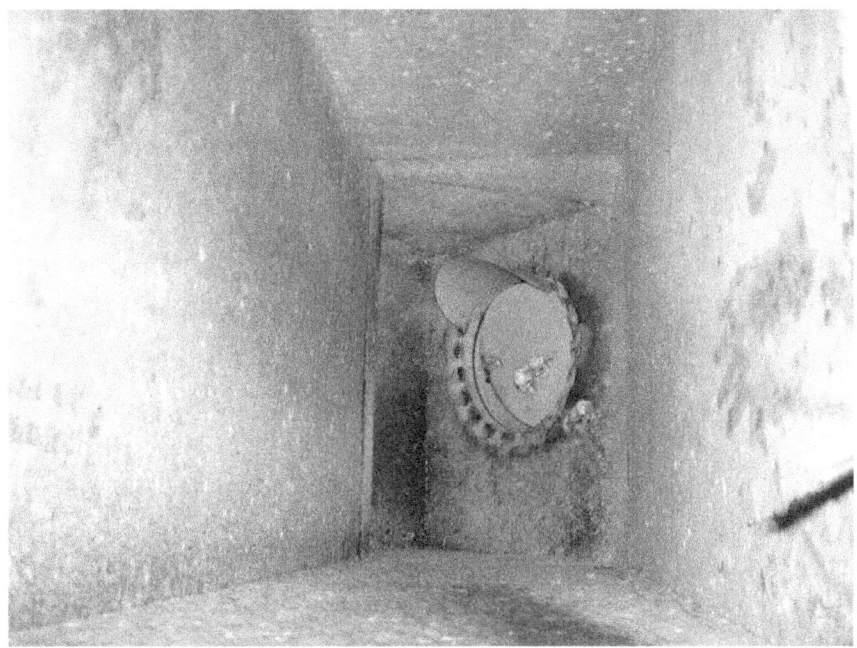

Figure 38. Inside supply duct after fan in AHU-4, June 2011.

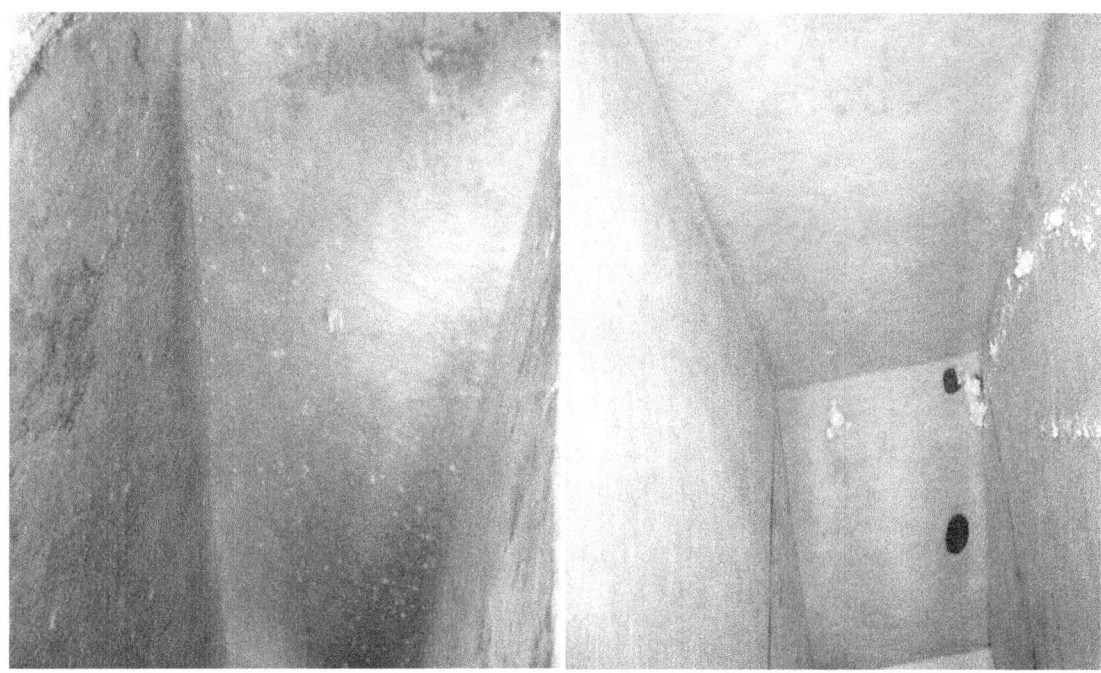

Figure 39. Inside supply duct immediately after fan, June 2011.
a) AHU- 4.   b) AHU-2 (light spots are sealant foam).

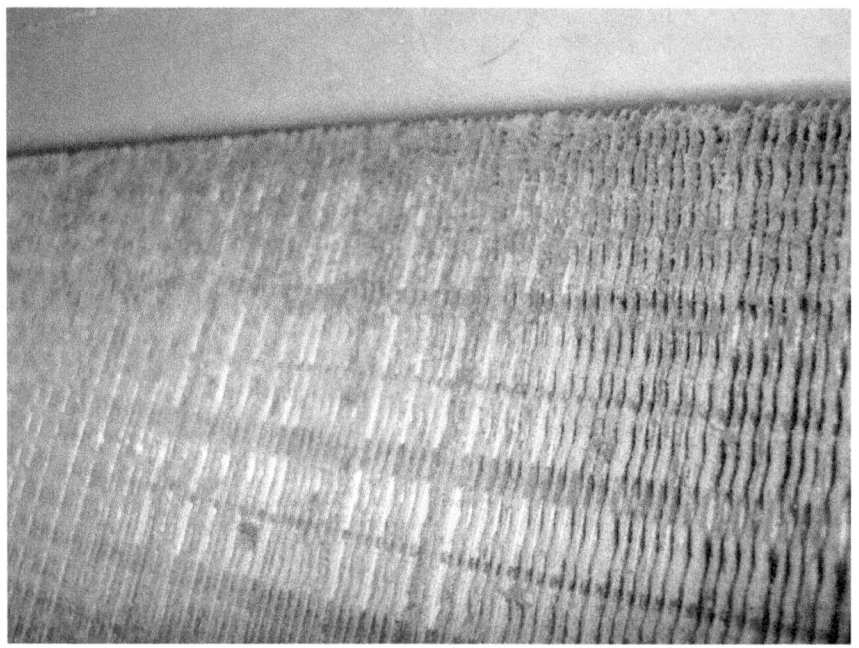

Figure 40. Cooling coil in AHU-3, June 2011.

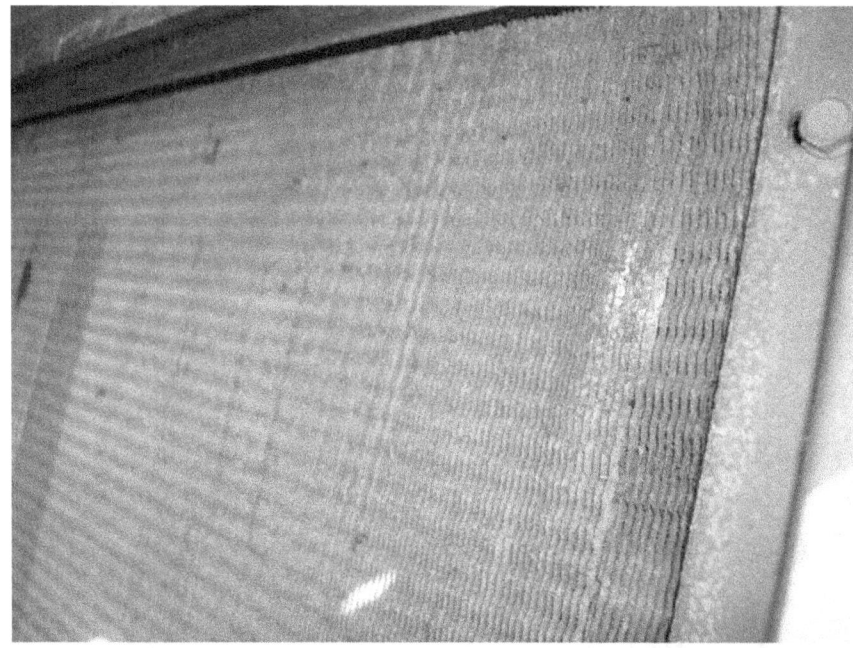

Figure 41. Cooling coil in AHU-4, June 2011.

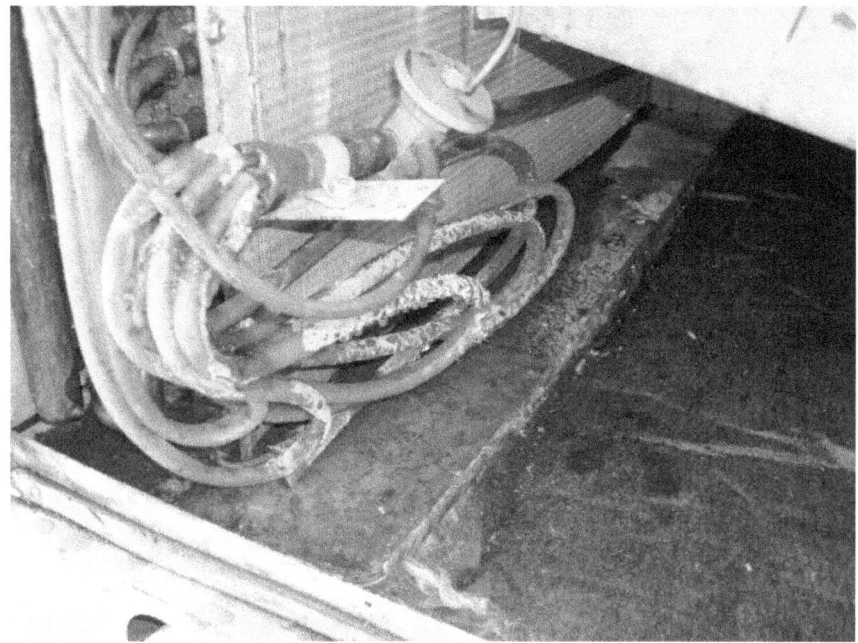

Figure 42. Inside of AHU-1, June 2011.

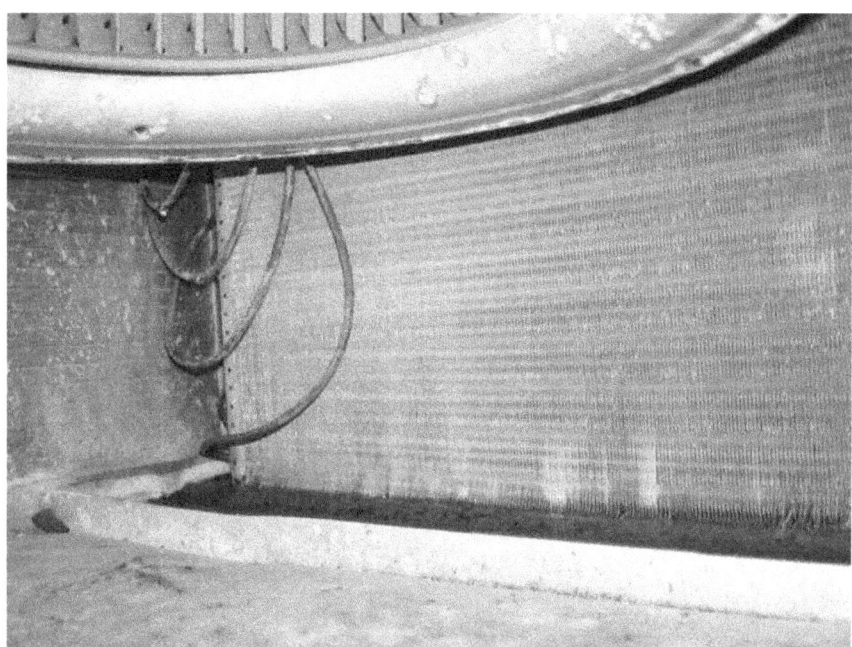

Figure 43. Inside of AHU-2, June 2011.

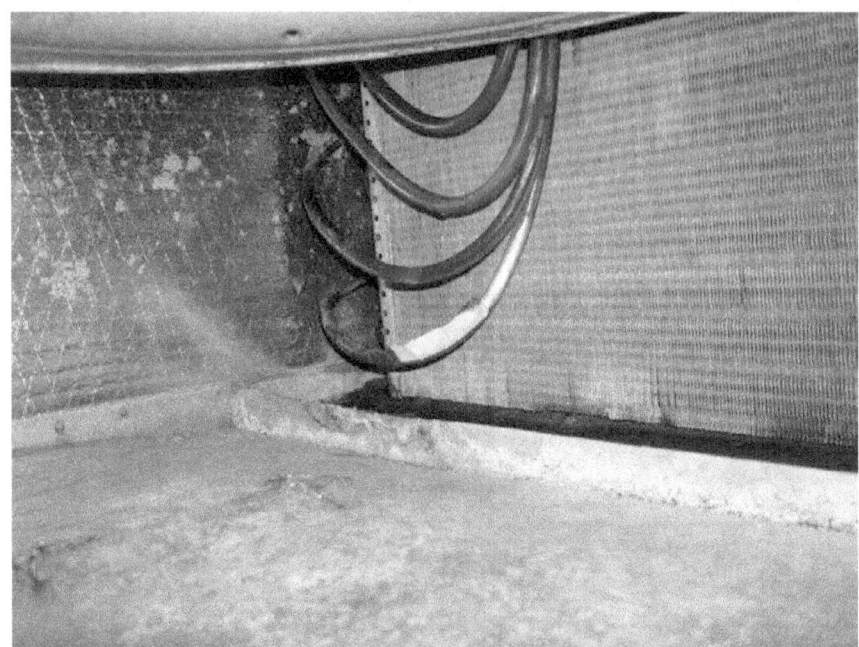

Figure 44. Inside of AHU-3, June 2011.

ACKNOWLEDGEMENTS AND AVAILABILITY OF REPORT

The Respiratory Disease Hazard Evaluation and Technical Assistance Program (RDHETAP) of NIOSH conducts field investigations of possible health hazards in the workplace. These investigations are conducted under the authority of Section 20(a)(6) of the Occupational Safety and Health (OSH) Act of 1970, 29 U.S.C. 669(a)(6), or Section 501(a)(11) of the Federal Mine Safety and Health Act of 1977, 30 U.S.C. 951(a)(11), which authorizes the Secretary of Health and Human Services, following a written request from any employers or authorized representative of employees, to determine whether any substance normally found in the place of employment has potentially toxic effects in such concentrations as used or found.

Mention of any company or product does not constitute endorsement by NIOSH. In addition, citations to websites external to NIOSH do no constitute NIOSH endorsement of the sponsoring organizations or their programs or products. Furthermore, NIOSH is not responsible for the content of these websites. All Web addresses referenced in this document were accessible as of the publication date.

RDHETAP also provides, upon request, technical and consultative assistance to federal, state, and local agencies; labor; industry; and other groups or individuals to control occupational health hazards and to prevent related trauma and disease.

This report was prepared by Rachel Bailey, Chris Piacitelli, Stephen Martin, Jr., Jean Cox-Ganser of RDHETAP. Site visit was conducted by Rachel Bailey and Chris Piacitelli. Industrial hygiene field assistance was provided by an environmental specialist from the local county health department. Desktop publishing was performed by Tia McClelland of RDHETAP. The authors thank Kathleen Kreiss and Nicole Edwards for their thoughtful review of this report.

Copies of this report have been sent to employee and management representatives at the accounting firm, the local and state health departments, and the OSHA Regional Office. This report is not copyrighted and may be freely reproduced. The report may be viewed and printed at www.cdc.gov/niosh/hhe/. Copies may be purchased from the National Technical Information Service (NTIS) at 5825 Port Royal Road, Springfield, Virginia 22161.